COPING
WITH
PEDIATRIC
ILLNESS

Coping

with

Pediatric

Illness

edited by
Charles E. Hollingsworth, M.D.

Child Psychiatrist
Ventura County Mental Health Services

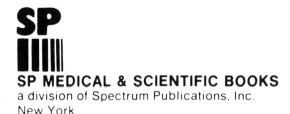

SP MEDICAL & SCIENTIFIC BOOKS
a division of Spectrum Publications, Inc.
New York

SPECTRUM PUBLICATIONS, INC.
175-20 Wexford Terrace
Jamaica, NY 11432

Library of Congress Cataloging in Publication Data
Main entry under title:

Coping with pediatric illness.

Includes index.
1. Pediatrics–Psychological aspects. 2. Sick children–Family relationships. 3. Physically handi-capped children–Psychology. 4. Medical personnel–Attitudes. I. Hollingsworth, Charles E. [DNLM:
1. Child psychology. 2. Chronic disease–Psychology.
3. Parent-child-relations. 4. Pediatrics. WS 200
c783]
RJ47.5.C67   1982   618.92'0001'9   82-10743
ISBN 0-89335-157-1

Printed in the United States of America

This volume is dedicated to George Tarjan who inspired me to become a child psychiatrist. Dr. Tarjan is President of the American Psychiatric Association, 1983-84.

CONTENTS

Contributors   ix

Preface   xi

1. The Use of Psychotropic Medication in the Pediatric Population   1
    Dennis P. Cantwell

2. Maternal Bonding and Infant Attachment   23
    Charles W. Ralston, and Mary J. O'Connor

3. Father-Infant Bonding and the Role of the Father in Child Rearing   41
    Charles E. Hollingsworth

4. The Pros and Cons of the Alternate Birth Room and
    the Dangers of Home Deliveries   45
    Katherine F. Carson

5. Nursing Considerations in the Alternate Birth Room,
    in the Normal Neonatal Nursery, and in Rooming-in   55
    Judith Trunecek

6. High-Risk Infant Follow-up   61
    Kristin Gist

7. The Role of the Psychologist in a Pediatric Setting   79
    Jack Wetter

8. Cognitive Skills and the Learning-disabled Youngster   89
    Nita Ferjo

9. The Role of Psychoeducation and the Educational Therapist in
    the Treatment of Emotionally Disturbed Children   105
    Jennifer L. Sokol

10. Recognition and Treatment of Child Sexual Abuse   115
    Roland Summit

11. The Psychological Effects of Genetic Disorders in Children and
     Their Parents   173
         Isabelle Leddet-Chevallier and Steve Funderburk

12. Emotional Impact of Hematology and Oncology Illnesses
     on the Child and Family   189
         M. M. "Sunny" Lindamood and Fran Wiley

13. The Psychosocial Aspects of Hemophilia   197
         Shelby L. Dietrich, Margaret A. Jaffe, and Margaret K. Reed

14. Psychological Considerations for the Cleft Palate Clinic and Team   201
         Yoshio Setoguchi and Patricia DuPont-Norton

15. Psychological Considerations in the Spinal Defects and
     Meningomyelocele Clinic   209
         Shirley T. Whiteman and Wendy S. Feldman

16. Psychological Effects of Duchenne's Muscular Dystrophy
     on Children and Their Families   229
         Irene S. Gilgoff

17. Psychotherapy for the Physically Disabled Child: Combining
     Interpretive/Supportive Therapy with Behavior Therapy   243
         Claude Amarnick

18. A Parent of a Disabled Child Looks at a Hospital and Its Services   253
         Linda Jefferson

Index   261

CONTRIBUTORS

Claude Amarnick, D. O.
Beth Israel Medical Center
New York, New York

Dennis Cantwell, M.D.
Joseph Campbell Professor of
  Child Psychiatry
Director of Residency Training in
  Child Psychiatry
UCLA Neuropsychiatric Institute
School of Medicine
University of California,
  Los Angeles

Katherine F. Carson, M.D.
Department of Obstetrics and
  Gynecology
Donald N. Sharp Memorial Hospital
San Diego, California

Shelby Dietrich, M.D.
Hemophilia Rehabilitation Center
Department of Pediatrics
Orthopaedic Hospital
Los Angeles, California

Patricia DuPont-Norton, L.C.S.W.
Department of Clinical Social Work
UCLA Hospital and Clinics
University of California,
  Los Angeles

Wendy Feldman, M.S.W.
Medical Social Worker
Department of Social Work
Orthopaedic Hospital
Los Angeles, California

Nita Ferjo, Ph.D.
Coordinator of Educational
  Consultants
Child Outpatient Department
UCLA Neuropsychiatric Institute
Los Angeles, California

Steve Funderburk, M.D.
Mental Retardation and Child
  Psychiatry Program and Division
  of Medical Genetics
Department of Psychiatry
School of Medicine
University of California,
  Los Angeles

Irene S. Gilgoff, M.D.
Department of Pediatrics
Rancho Los Amigos Hospital
Orthopaedic Hospital and
  USC Medical Center
Downey, California
Los Angeles, California

Kristin Gist, M.S.
Neonatal Follow-up Project
Children's Hospital and Health Center
San Diego, California

Charles E. Hollingsworth, M.D.
Child Psychiatrist and Pediatrician
Ventura County Mental Health
  Services
Ventura, California

Margaret A. Jaffe, M.S.W.
Hemophilia Rehabilitation Center
Department of Pediatrics
Orthopaedic Hospital
Los Angeles, California

Linda Jefferson, R.N.
Children's Hospital and
   Health Center
San Diego, California

Isabelle Leddet-Chevallier, M.D.
Centre Hospitalier Universitaire
Tours Cedex, France

Sunny Lindamood, L.C.S.W.
Department of Pediatrics
UCLA Hospital and Clinics
University of California,
   Los Angeles

Mary J. O'Connor, Ph.D.
Assistant Adjunct Professor of
   Pediatrics
School of Medicine
University of California,
   Los Angeles
Assistant Research Psychologist
UCLA Neuropsychiatric Institute
Los Angeles, California

Charles W. Ralston, M.D.
Fellow, Division of Child
   Development
Department of Pediatrics
School of Medicine
University of California,
   Los Angeles

Margaret K. Reed, M.S.W.
Hemophilia Rehabilitation Center
Department of Pediatrics
Orthopaedic Hospital
Los Angeles, California

Yoshio Setoguchi, M.D.
Adjunct Professor of Medicine
Department of Pediatrics
Medical Director, Child Amputee
   Prosthetics Project
School of Medicine
University of California,
   Los Angeles

Jennifer L. Sokol, M.Ed.
Educational Therapy Coordinator
Thalians Community Mental Health
   Center
Cedars-Sinai Medical Center
Los Angeles, California

Roland Summit, M.D.
Assistant Professor of Psychiatry
School of Medicine
University of California,
   Los Angeles
Head Physician, Community
   Consultation Service
Harbor — UCLA Medical Center
Torrance, California

Judith Trunecek, R.N., B.S.N.
Managing Coordinator, Nursery
Donald N. Sharp Memorial
   Community Hospital
San Diego, California

Jack Wetter, Ed.D.
Director, Psychological Services
Marion Davies Children's Clinic
UCLA Center for the Health
   Sciences
Adjunct Assistant Professor
School of Medicine
University of California,
   Los Angeles

Shirley Whiteman, M.D., F.A.A.P.
Pediatric Coordinator
Spina Bifida Clinic
Department of Pediatrics
Orthopaedic Hospital
Los Angeles, California

Fran Wiley, R.N.
Division of Hematology and
   Oncology
Department of Pediatrics
UCLA Center for the Health
   Sciences
University of California,
   Los Angeles

Preface

Coping with Pediatric Illness is a companion book to *Pediatric Consultation Liaison Psychiatry* which was written at the same time and edited by this editor. *Coping with Pediatric Illness* contains chapters by leading experts in the fields of child psychiatry and pediatrics. The chapters which they contribute are greatly appreciated by those of us who work with physically ill children and their families.

This book begins with an overview of the use of psychotropic medication in pediatrics by Dennis Cantwell, MD, who was my mentor at the UCLA Neuropsychiatric Institute during my training as an adult and child psychiatrist and as a fully trained pediatrician. Next, we focus on infant development, maternal-infant bonding, father-infant bonding, pros and cons of the alternate birth rooms, nursing considerations in the alternate birth room, and the high-risk infant follow-up project. Then, we emphasize the role of the psychologist in pediatrics, the cognitive skills of the learning disabled child, and the role of psychoeducation and the educational therapist in the treatment of emotionally disturbed children.

Dr. Roland Summit's chapter on the "Recognition and Treatment of Child Sexual Abuse," which is sure to become a "classic," is featured in *Coping with Pediatric Illness* because I felt that everyone who works with children will benefit from his insight, his explanation of the dynamics of the perpetrators, victims, and their families, and his discussion of the magnitude of the problem.

This chapter is followed by two which focus specifically on the psychological considerations of genetic disorders and the overwhelming psychological impact of hematologic and oncologic illnesses on children and their families.

Next, the nation's leading experts share their years of experience in relating their advice and recommendations for assisting parents and children coping with cleft palate, spinal defects, and muscular dystrophy. These three chapters contain information on new advances in the treatment of these conditions and highlight some optimism regarding the psychological impact of these ailments.

The conclusion of the book includes two chapters which emphasize the needs of the disabled child—Dr. Claude Amarnick's insightful chapter, "Psychotherapy for the Physically Disabled Child," and Linda Jefferson's sensitive and caring chapter, "The Parent of a Disabled Child Looks at the Hospital and Its Services."

Those persons who work in child psychiatry and who provide emotional support to children and their families will benefit from using *Coping with Pediatric*

Illness in conjunction with *Pediatric Consultation Liaison Psychiatry*. I believe that pediatricians and pediatric nurses will find *Coping with Pediatric Illness* a must on their reading list this year. Physically ill children and their families appreciate caregivers who are humane and caring, as gentle as possible, and well-read regarding the latest and most up-to-date procedures, techniques, and treatment, including child mental health advances. These two books were written to enable all of us to better cope with the tragedy of severe illness in our children.

Charles E. Hollingsworth, MD

COPING
WITH
PEDIATRIC
ILLNESS

The Use of Psychotropic Medication in the Pediatric Population

Dennis P. Cantwell

This chapter will review the use of psychotropic medication in the pediatric population. A historical perspective will be given first, then general principles regarding the use of psychopharmacologic agents with children will be reviewed, and finally the author will present his personal view on the use of psychopharmacologic agents with specific disorders in childhood.

HISTORICAL PERSPECTIVE

Without question the introduction of psychopharmacologic agents in the United States in the early 1950s drastically altered the clinical practice of psychiatry with *adult patients*. Moreover, as more has become known about the biological actions of psychotropic drugs, new research areas have opened up with adult psychiatric disorders. Prior to the introduction of phenothiazines and other major tranquilizers in 1952, many chronic schizophrenic patients remained hospitalized in large state institutions because of their inability to be managed in an outpatient setting. The benefits in these major psychiatric disorders that have accrued from the development of the major tranquilizers has led to a decrease in state hospital populations and to an increased quality of life for these previously chronic patients.

Major affective disorders, in the United States—bipolar illness, characterized by episodes of mania and depression, and unipolar illness, characterized by episodes of depression—remain a major public health problem. The lifetime morbidity risk for males for the development of a major depressive episode is between 10 and 12 percent. The same figure for females is between 20 and 25 percent (Klein et al., 1980). Prior to the introduction of the monoamine oxidase inhibitors and the tricyclic antidepressants in the late 1950s, treatment of major depressive disorders and of mania was very difficult. Introduction of the major antidepressant drugs and lithium changed the outlook for patients with major affective disorders. Moreover, an investigation of the biological actions of the tricyclic antidepressants and the monoamine oxidase inhibitors led to the formulation of various theories of biogenic amine metabolism and their role in major depressive disorders. This area of research—biological correlates of major affective disorders in adult psychiatric patients—probably is the single most productive area of biological research in adult psychiatry. The introduction of lithium also added a new dimension to psychopharmacologic practice with adults. Lithium was introduced as an antimanic, effective for the manic phase of bipolar affective disorder. However, over time the evidence seems to indicate that lithium is not only clearly effective for the manic phase, but is also effective for the depressive phase in some patients, and may also exert a prophylactic effect on the development of subsequent manic and depressive episodes. Thus, the last 20 to 30 years have witnessed major advances in the use of psychopharmacologic agents with *adults* with psychiatric disorders.

The use of psychopharmacologic agents with *children* actually predates these developments with adults by many years. If one begins as a starting point with Bradley's classical studies of amphetamines in Providence, Rhode Island, in the late 1930s (Bradley, 1937), pediatric psychopharmacology can be seen to have a 20-year head start on the major developments in adult psychopharmacology. However, neither practice nor research with psychiatric disorders of childhood has been as affected by the use of psychotropic medication as is the case with adult psychiatry. There are a variety of reasons why this is true. As has been pointed out elsewhere (Cantwell, 1978), in many child psychiatric training centers psychopharmacologic therapy is not emphasized as a primary therapeutic modality. Child psychiatry in the United States did not grow up as a purely medical discipline. Rather, the roots of child psychiatry in the United States are in the child guidance clinics of the 1920s. As a result, many of the people involved in training in child psychiatry did not themselves have adequate exposure to the use of psychopharmacologic agents in their training years. Thus, they did not use them in their practice and, when they trained future practitioners, did not consider them when discussing differential therapy for patients. It is the author's opinion that if a trainee is not exposed to and does not become comfortable with the use of psychoactive medication in training years, it is unlikely that he will make significant use of them in later years in practice.

Aside from the training issue, it must also be recognized that there is a vocal antimedication body in the United States. The proponents of this antimedication viewpoint espouse the view that the use of psychoactive agents with children is putting children in "chemical strait-jackets." In their view, psychopharmacologic agents are used to control bright, active, exuberant children who come into conflict with our system of education. Most of this antimedication viewpoint is found in the public media. Very often it is tied in with certain "magical cures" that have little in the way of scientific validity behind them. It is true that serious thought must be given to long-term use of psychotropic medication with children. However, it is a serious mistake to think that proper use of psychopharmacologic agents produces controlled robots. The decision of whether to use a psychoactive drug with a psychiatrically disordered child should be based on the severity of the child's condition, what is known about its untreated outcome, and what is known about the clinical efficacy and safety of the particular medication one is considering using. This is a medical decision and should be made by physicians, not a philosophical one to be made by philosophers.

Finally, there are some special factors relating to the fact that the child is a developing organism that affect both clinical practice and research. The most important ones are: diagnostic factors, biological factors, assessment factors, and family factors.

Diagnostic classification of psychiatric disorders in childhood is in a much more rudimentary state than it is with adult psychiatric disorders. A considerable amount is known about the well-studied adult psychiatric disorders, such as schizophrenic disorders, the anxiety disorders, and the affective disorders. Thus, research has proceeded at a much faster pace regarding psychopharmacologic treatment of these disorders. Until very recently, the issue of psychiatric diagnosis in childhood was one considered very lightly, if it was considered at all. Until the introduction of the *Diagnostic and Statistical Manual (DSM-III)* by the American Psychiatric Association in 1980, there did not exist a classification system comprehensive enough to cover the major psychiatric disorders of childhood with operational criteria to insure reliability of diagnosis and some homogeneity of patient populations. Thus, previous studies have used terms like "minimal brain dysfunction," "hyperkinetic child," and "hyperactive child" to describe what is reportedly the same condition. However, with the lack of operational criteria and confusion about the terminology, this undoubtedly meant that the same children were described by different people with different terms, and different children were being described by different investigators with the same terms. This diagnostic heterogeneity of patient populations leads to difficulties in interpretations of psychotropic drug studies from center to center.

In contrast to the adult psychiatric patient, the child still is an immature developing organism. This has relevance to developmental changes in symptom patterns as well as in biological functions. With regard to developmental changes in symptom patterns, the same behaviors may have different causes and meanings at different ages and thus may respond differently to the same drug at different ages. Moreover, as the child grows older, certain symptoms, such as excess motor activity, may diminish or disappear in adolescence, yet the child still manifests certain symptomatology of his original disorder. Thus, if one were monitoring one symptom, such as activity level, it would seem that as the child grew older medication would no longer be necessary, but what is actually happening is that the wrong symptoms are being monitored at a later age. Since children are still developing, absorption and detoxification mechanisms may differ from child to child, as they may develop at different rates in different children. Thus, the same dosage of a drug may lead to different blood levels from child to child. This, in turn, might lead to differences in drug response for children of the same age, the same body weight, and the same psychiatric disorder. Side effects may also be related to chronological age and maturational level. Younger children, who have a more limited repertoire of behavior than older children, react in a relatively nonspecific manner to a wide variety of factors, including drug toxicity.

Family factors probably play a larger role in drug treatment of children than they do of psychiatrically disordered adults. In general, children are brought for psychiatric evaluation not because of their own wishes, but because their behavior is bothersome to the parents, to the school, or to both. Moreover, children must live directly in the family setting, in contrast to adults, and thus are probably more affected by a disordered parent-child interaction and other family factors. The parents' attitude toward the use of medication for their child may also be a crucial factor. Parents obviously are the ones to administer the drug to younger children, and if they feel the medication is not effective or should not be used with their child, then it may simply not be given. Reliance is usually made very heavily on reports from the parents on the effectiveness or noneffectiveness of any drug as well. The parents' view of whether the drug is working may be clouded by their views toward the use of medication.

The physician's manner of presenting the use of medication to the family also probably plays a role in whether or not the medication is considered to be effective. Unfortunately, many physicians present the use of psychotropic drugs to the parents as an "either/or phenomenon," that is, drugs are not considered until other modalities are tried and found not to be effective. The attitude of "if nothing else works, we'll try medication" may subtly influence the way parents assess the therapeutic value of any medication.

With regard to the research literature on the effectiveness of psychoactive drugs, certain things have to be pointed out that are almost truisms. How the dosage is determined in any particular study may determine whether the drug is judged effective or not. Fixed dosage studies may offer information on certain pharmacokinetic properties of medication, but they may also lead to inadequate dosage levels for an individual child. The methods used to assess drug effect in a research study and in practice is also an important issue. The physician's observations of change in an office setting is the most inadequate way of monitoring drug effect in children, particularly in younger children. Children behave differently in different settings, and a comprehensive picture must be obtained on the effect of medication in different settings in order to truly assess the effect of drugs. Thus, standardized rating scales are available for completion by parents and teachers, and they are more effective and reliable in assessing positive and negative effects of psychopharmacologic agents than are anecdotal reports or unsystematic observations.

It would be helpful if laboratory measures could be used to assess drug effect both in practice and in research settings. However, in a great majority of cases reliable, meaningful laboratory tests have not been used to assess drug effects with most of the psychotropic drugs used with children. Finally, from the research standpoint, it is mandatory that the effectiveness of any drug for any disorder be established by a properly controlled and analyzed study. This requires operational diagnostic criteria to insure as much homogeneity as possible of the patient population, random assignment to drug and placebo categories, proper monitoring of medications, reliable and standardized measures of assessment, and proper statistical analysis. While this would seem to be an obvious statement, there are many published studies in the child psychopharmacology area that do not meet minimal criteria of scientific acceptability. However, over the last ten years this picture has improved greatly, especially with certain psychiatric disorders in children, such as attention deficit disorder with hyperactivity.

GENERAL PRINCIPLES OF PEDIATRIC PSYCHOPHARMACOLOGY

There are some general principles that apply no matter what drug one is using and no matter what disorder is being treated. The general principles involve: (1) a comprehensive diagnostic evaluation of the child; (2) proper baseline assessments of target symptoms; (3) involvement of the family; (4) involvement of the school; (5) selection of the drug; (6) titration of medication; (7) monitoring of medication; (8) drug-free trial and reevaluation (Cantwell, 1979; Cantwell and Carlson, 1978).

Comprehensive Diagnostic Evaluation of the Child

Evaluation should include a detailed interview with the parents about the child, a detailed psychiatric interview of the child, physical and neurological examinations, obtaining information from the school, observing appropriate laboratory studies (including psychological tests), and interviews with the parents about family structure, family dynamics, family interaction, and the greater psychosocial environment of the child. The interview with the child and the interview with the parents have been described in detail elsewhere (Cantwell,

1975), and only the high points will briefly be mentioned here. In recent years, semistructured interviews, such as the K-SADS and the DICA, have been developed to standardize the history-taking procedure for the psychiatric evaluation of children much in the same way as the DIS and the SADS have done with adults. This plus the advent of the *DSM-III* diagnostic system, which uses operational diagnostic criteria for each psychiatric disorder, promise to lead to more diagnostic homogeneity in patient populations. It is important to note that in the interview with the parents one must have a systematic coverage of all possible behavior manifestations of psychiatric disorders of childhood. It is important that the parents be given an opportunity to tell their own story in their own way. However, at some point a systematic coverage must be made of all areas of the child's functioning. This is because the parents may bring in the child for one set of symptoms, such as short attention span, impulsive behavior, etc., while the child may manifest more severe pathology, such as severe depression and suicidal ideation, that the parents may not be aware of or that they may not consider to be as important.

The interview with the child, likewise, must be a systematic one. The tradition in child psychiatric interviewing has often been one of a play interview that is not geared toward obtaining symptomatic information. However, symptomatic information can be obtained from children above the age of seven or so, and an attempt must be made to complement what is obtained from the parental interview and from material obtained from the school. During the interview with the child, two types of information are obtained: information obtained verbally from the child (either spontaneously or in response to direct questions) and observations made of the child during the interview. Some attempt should be made to assess those areas that are presented by parents and teachers as difficulties. Thus, if a child is referred for having short attention span, some attempt should be made during the interview to test the child's attention span and distractability. It is helpful to record the systematic observations made during the interview on a standardized scale that one can then use for future reference in monitoring drug treatment if medication is indicated and initiated. Information obtained from the school and information obtained in the interview with the parent and the interview with the child will generally contain the sources that lead to the diagnosis of a specific type of psychiatric disorder. It is only rarely that a physical examination, neurological examination, and laboratory studies contribute to the diagnosis of a *specific* psychiatric disorder in childhood, although they may add information that is important in individual cases.

In the physical examination, stress should be placed on a screening of all body systems, at least by interrogation of parent and child. The central nervous system should be particularly emphasized, and a screening neurological examination should be carried out. Baseline height, weight, blood pressure, and pulse should be recorded. The pediatric psychopharmacologic section of the ECDEU

(Guy, 1976) package offers very helpful materials in this area. From the stand-point of laboratory studies, it is important to recognize that younger children do not like blood tests, and they really only need to be done if there are clear clinical indications that the child may have some specific physical or neuro-logical problem or if toxic effects have developed as a result of the use of some medication. A baseline screening battery, such as a complete blood count, urinalysis, and SMA-12, is probably all that needs to be done initially. If there are no specific problems, either initially or that develop over time, the tests need to be repeated only at rare intervals.

Proper Baseline Assessments

All psychotropic drugs affect multiple bodily functions. The ones that are most important in the management of psychiatric disorders in childhood include: activity level, cognitive function, academic achievement, behavior, per-sonality, mood, and the physiological systems of the body. Thus, it is important to have some assessment of all of these areas at baseline so that they can be monitored over time. Behavior rating scales have been developed by a variety of individuals to be completed by parents and teachers. These include such things as the Rutter parent and teacher questionnaire (Rutter, Graham, and Yule, 1970), the behavior problem checklist developed by Quay (1980), Conners' parent and teacher rating scale (Guy, 1976), and other specific scales. The Conners parent and teacher rating scale seem to have been used the most in psychopharmacologic studies and are part of the ECDEU pediatric psychophar-macology package.

The physician's clinical global impression is also a quite useful rating. Side-effect rating scales to be completed by parent, patient, and physician are also part of the ECDEU package and should be completed at baseline, since it is important to recognize that some behaviors, which may be side effects of certain drugs, may actually be present at baseline.

Since all psychotropic drugs are going to affect cognitive function, it is impor-tant to have some psychoeducational assessment, which should include, as a minimum, assessment of general intelligence and of academic achievement. There are a variety of tests of cognitive function that have found some use in some drug studies, such as: the reaction time, the continuous performance task, the paired-associate learning task, short-term memory task, studies of discrimin-ation learning, the matching familiar figures test, the Bender and Frostig tests, the Illinois test of psycholinguistic abilities, and the Porteus maze (Aman, 1978). Some of these have found more utility than others in drug studies.

Certain drugs may have a cognitive dulling effect and, if no measure of cog-nitive function is obtained and only behavioral measures are monitored, one may observe an improvement in behavior at the expense of a dulling of cognitive function. This is especially true with retarded individuals.

Family Involvement

Once the comprehensive diagnostic evaluation has been completed and once the diagnostic formulation has been made and proper baseline assessments have been completed, the physician then makes a decision as to whether or not a trial of some psychoactive medication is warranted. This decision should be based on the severity of the condition, its untreated natural history, what is known about the efficacy and safety of certain drugs in treating it, and whether or not there are specific contraindications to psychoactive drug usage in this particular case. Once the decision has been made to use the psychotropic medication, the next step is involvement of the parents and the child in the treatment process. A neglected part of the use of psychopharmacologic agents is trying to help the child understand the nature of their difficulties and how the use of the medication is intended to help the child help himself.

A similar type of counseling must be done with the parents. In general, it is likely that with an individual child one will have to change either the type of medication or the dosage in order to get the optimal effect of the optimal drug for each child. The physician should prepare the parents for this, and he should explain in great detail exactly what the positive and negative effects of the medication might be. Since the physician will be requiring regular parental reports as a help in assessing drug effect, it is important to know what expectations the parents have about what the drug will do and what it will not do. If the parents have certain magical expectations about what the medication will do that are not fulfilled, they will report that the medication is ineffective, even when it may be doing exactly what physiologically it was intended to do. Parents should be encouraged to observe their child carefully for both positive and possible negative effects of the drug.

Involvement of the School

Good rapport must be obtained with the school in order to properly manage a child on any psychotropic drugs. It is important to make direct contact with the child's teacher in person or by phone to enlist her cooperation. The emphasis of her importance as an observer who can make judgments that other people are not in a position to make should be stressed. For example, certain medications, such as stimulants for attention deficit disorder, are prescribed so that they are effective only during the school day and are not at an effective blood level when the child returns home from school. Thus, the teacher may be the only person to see the child on an effective dose of medication. Moreover, she is likely to see the child in a setting that stresses his symptomatology. She also has a ready-made control group with whom to compare the child's behavior both on and off medication. Relying solely on the reports from parents or on his own observations, the physician is likely to underestimate both the positive and negative effects of the medication.

Selection of the Drug

Selection of a drug to be used in the treatment of any psychiatric disorder in childhood should be based on solid clinical evidence in the literature of its efficacy and safety. In general, there are three levels of indications for drugs, depending on the level of studies that have been done. The first level is a *definite* indication. A definite indication means that there is a substantial number of double-blind, properly controlled and properly analyzed studies that have been done with this drug with this particular disorder to indicate that it is indeed effective for the condition to be treated.

The second level could be called *possible* indications. Possible indications occur when there are not enough double-blind studies to suggest that the particular drug is definitely indicated for a particular disorder. However, there are a number of *open* studies that suggest that the drug *might* be effective. Open studies are obviously more useful in chronic conditions, which do not have spontaneous remissions. For example, open studies of antidepressants in the treatment of depression are not all that useful, since depression is an episodic disorder with spontaneous remission. Thus, if all patients are treated and there is a response, one cannot tell whether the response is due to the medication or whether it is a spontaneous remission or a placebo effect.

Another way a drug can be considered as a possible indication is if the known physiological action of the drug affects mechanisms that are thought to play a central role in the disorder. For example, it is well known that stimulants are effective for a large percentage of children who have attention deficit disorder with hyperactivity. It seems that the medication primarily affects the attentional process in this disorder. Attention deficit disorder without hyperactivity also is characterized by significant problems with attention in the *absence* of the motoric overactivity. One could hypothesize that stimulants might be effective for this disorder as well. To date there are no double-blind, placebo-controlled studies to support or reject this hypothesis, but stimulants could be considered a possible indication for this disorder.

The third level is a *nonindication*. This simply means that there is no evidence that the drug is effective for a particular condition.

Once the class of drugs is selected (e.g., stimulants for attention deficit disorder with hyperactivity), as a general rule a familiar and trusted drug should be the first choice. This is because there is much more evidence over time for drugs that have been around for many years than for drugs that have been on the market for a shorter period of time. The initial dosage of any medication should probably be the smallest dosage or, possibly, even half of it. The knowledge of the duration of action of any medication is obviously necessary to know how often it should be prescribed. Some drugs can be prescribed on a once-a-day basis, others on a two- or three-times-a-day basis, depending on how long the physician wishes the medication to be effective. Medications that do not develop significant blood levels over time (such as methylphenidate) have to be prescribed differently from those that do (such as the phenothiazines).

Titration and Monitoring of Medication

The next process is to titrate the medication until clinical improvement is noted or until side effects occur that necessitate continuation of the medication. For most conditions and for most drugs, there are very few laboratory or other measures against which medication can be titrated. In general practice, the physician will use clinical judgment based on information obtained from the parents, from the school, and from direct observation of the child. If improvement does occur after a medication has started, then the patient needs to be monitored at regular intervals. The same ratings of behavior that were taken initially at baseline should be made at regular intervals, including information from the parents, from the teacher, and the child himself about any positive and/or negative effects. Any other appropriate measures (e.g., measures of learning, depressive affect, anxiety, height, weight, etc.) should be done on a regular basis.

For most drugs and for most disorders there are *rough* guidelines that one can use for optimal dosage of an individual drug based on milligrams of drug per kilogram of body weight. However, it is well to recognize that an individual child may need more medication than would be expected on the basis of body weight. There are large individual differences in blood levels of medication for comparable dosages of the same drug in children of the same body weight.

Drug-Free Trial and Reevaluation

In many cases children who are on chronic psychoactive medication should be given a drug-free trial at some time during the course of a year. This will vary from drug to drug and from condition to condition. The best way of doing this is probably to substitute a placebo, without letting the child, the teacher, or the parent know that medication has been withdrawn, and determine if there is any deterioration of learning and behavior. However, this method is not always available to the practicing physician. Thus, in many cases it is best to let the child start a new school year in a new class with a new teacher in a medication-free state. After several weeks in the new class, baseline ratings can be obtained and compared with those obtained at the end of the previous school year when the child was on medication. If it appears that the child no longer needs treatment, he can be monitored closely to see if behavior or learning deteriorate over time. There is no good way other than clinical judgment for determining when a psychoactive medication should be discontinued completely. Medication should be stopped only when the clinical picture indicates that a child no longer requires it, not because he reaches a certain age or any other idiosyncratic factor.

SPECIFIC USES OF PSYCHOPHARMACOLOGIC AGENTS IN CHILDREN

A complete discussion of the use of specific psychopharmacologic agents with each of the psychiatric disorders of childhood is beyond the scope of this chapter. However, there are up-to-date reviews that can be found in several recent books (Werry, 1978; Klein et al., 1980). The goal of any psychopharmacologic treatment with any child will be the promotion of more normal patterns of maturation and development. It is important to recognize that in most cases children with psychiatric disorders will be treated with other forms of therapy *in addition to, not instead of*, drug therapy. The use of psychopharmacologic agents with children should not be used as an either/or phenomenon.

The second important principle is that any psychotropic drug affects multiple target functions. Thus, these need to be assessed in every child whatever the drug being used and whatever the disorder being treated. The most important functions include activity level, cognitive function and performance, academic achievement, behavior, personality, mood, and the body's physiological systems (especially the autonomic, peripherial, and central nervous systems). What follows then is a brief review of the various psychotropic drugs in common use and their definitie and possible indication. Specific references to support these statements can be found in several recent, very comprehensive reviews (Werry, 1978; Klein et al., 1980).

Stimulants

The only definite indication for the use of stimulants with children is *attention deficit disorder with hyperactivity*. This is the *DSM-III* term for the condition that was previously called "hyperkinetic reaction of childhood," "hyperactive child syndrome," and, unofficially, "minimal brain dysfunction." It is characterized by symptoms of inattention, overactivity, and impulsiveness. It is more common in boys, begins early in life, and appears to be a rather chronic condition. There is a significant number of double-blind studies to suggest that about 75 percent of children with this disorder have a positive response to central nervous stimulants such as methylphenidate, the amphetamines, and magnesium pemoline.

There are five conditions that *might* be considered possible indications for the use of stimulants. Two of these are *attention deficit disorder without hyperactivity* and *attention deficit disorder residual state*. Both of these are newly described conditions in *DSM-III*. Attention deficit disorder without hyperactivity is characterized by inattention and impulsiveness without motoric overactivity symptoms. Attention deficit disorder residual state applies to adolescents and adults who manifested attention deficit disorder with hyperactivity in childhood and no longer meet the essential criteria, but who still have difficulties relating to their original disorder. Paul Wender (personal communication) has done a number of studies with attention deficit disorder residual state and has found that the response to stimulants that one finds in childhood still is obtained with many adults with this disorder. The author has likewise found attention deficit disorder without hyperactivity to be responsive to stimulants.

Conduct disorders are characterized by repeated violations of society norms or individuals' rights. There is a large literature on the use of stimulants with conduct-disordered children dating back to Hill's original study in 1937 (Hill, 1947). The question of whether conduct-disordered children who do respond to stimulants are actually grown up ADD children with a significant amount of antisocial symptomatology is very much a possibility. At least one study by Maletsky (1974) does suggest that that is true.

Specific developmental disorders, such as reading disorder, are in some cases characterized by significant problems with attention difficulties. *Theoretically*, stimulants might be effective for some children with these types of problems, although the data to support this are lacking. Finally, there are some *mentally retarded children* and *children with pervasive developmental disorders* (such as those with infantile autism) who likewise present with symptoms of inattentiveness, low frustration tolerance, impulsiveness, and hyperactivity. In some cases the secondary symptoms *may* be benefited by the use of stimulants to the same extent that attention deficit disorder with hyperactivity (without mental retardation or pervasive developmental disorder) is benefited.

There should be some caution in the use of stimulants with the retarded with symptoms of attention deficit disorder. There is some indication, at least in some cases, that while behavioral improvement may occur, the stimulants may have a negative effect on learning because the nature of the attention span deficit in the retarded is significantly different than it is in the nonretarded, and the stimulants may in fact lead to a more fixed attention span (Aman, 1978).

Antidepressants

There are only two definite indications for the current use of antidepressants in children. One is *enuresis* and the second is *attention deficit disorder with hyperactivity*. There are numerous double-blind, placebo-controlled studies to suggest that antidepressants such as Tofranil are indeed effective for a substantial number of children with enuresis. However, the relapse rate once the drug is withdrawn is also quite high. The response rate is somewhat lower than can be achieved with a conditioning program such as the buzzer and pad, and the relapse rate to the conditioning program is lower. Thus, even though this is a definite indication in the sense that there are significant double-blind, controlled studies to attest to its effectiveness, the author's personal opinion is that the antidepressants should be used only if the conditioning program fails, or, the two might be used concurrently.

With attention deficit disorder with hyperactivity, the evidence does suggest that roughly the same percentage of children will have a positive response to antidepressants as to stimulants. However, the long-term use of antidepressants with attention deficit disorder with hyperactivity does not seem to be as good; the response does not seem to be as well maintained as it is with stimulants. Moreover, the antidepressants are potentially more toxic, particularly in the cardiotoxic area, than the stimulants and probably ought to be used only when a thorough trial with stimulants produces no response or produces side effects that are not tolerable.

The possible indications for the use of antidepressants in children include: *depression, conduct disorder, separation anxiety,* and the *specific developmental disorders.*

The question of depression in childhood is a very complex one and, until recently, a very much underinvestigated one. In the past, the most common view of depression in childhood was that when it did occur, it did not present with the clinical picture of depression as we know in adults. Rather, the depression was "masked" by a wide variety of other symptoms, which included such things as separation anxiety, conduct disorder, hyperactivity, enuresis, etc. The rationale for such a view often hinged on the fact that some of these children do get a positive response to antidepressants. Thus, the implication was that a response to a drug made the diagnosis, even in the absence of dysphoric mood, anhedonia, and other characteristic symptoms of depression as we know it in adults. This argument, of course, is quite circular. It is well known that antidepressants, like all psychotropic drugs, affect many functions, and a response to a particular psychotropic drug cannot be taken as an indication that a certain diagnosis is present.

Recently, there has been research in a number of centers—particularly in Los Angeles, Pittsburgh, and New York—to suggest that, indeed, there are children who do meet the criteria for depression as we know it in adults. Moreover, when antidepressants are used in the appropriate dosage to obtain a therapeutic blood level, they do get a positive response to antidepressants very much in line with the response that is found with depression in adults. Much more work, however, needs to be done in this area before one would consider this a definite indication.

Likewise, there are open-trial studies and at least one double-blind, controlled study to suggest that children with separation anxiety disorder with panic attacks also get a positive response to antidepressants, irrespective of the presence or severity of depressed mood. The mechanism for this response is probably different from that of the antidepressant response in that it is a rather immediate response, similar to that found with enuresis and attention deficit disorder with hyperactivity. More work needs to be done with this condition to replicate previous findings.

There is a relatively large literature on the use of antidepressants for the treatment of "masked depression," with such symptoms as conduct disorders and specific developmental disorders. These are all open-trial studies with many methodological flaws. However, they do suggest that a wide variety of symptoms may be improved by the use of antidepressants. It is hoped that future research will delineate more conclusively exactly which disorders respond to antidepressant usage in childhood and how, since antidepressants have proved to be such a valuable psychotropic agent with psychiatric disorders in adult life.

Antipsychotics (Major Tranquilizers)

The use of the terms "major tranquilizer" and "minor tranquilizer," while quite popular, is incorrect and potentially misleading, since it seems to indicate that the antianxiety agents, which are often called minor tranquilizers, are on a severity continuim with the major tranquilizers, often called antipsychotics. This is certainly not true, since their physiological action is fundamentally quite distinct. On the other hand, the use of the term "antipsychotic" can also be somewhat misleading, considering their use in children.

There are three conditions that can occur in childhood that could be considered definite indications for the use of antipsychotics (such as the phenothiazines); these are: *schizophrenia, mania,* and *Tourette's syndrome.* Schizophrenia as we know it in adults, characterized by formal thought disorder, blunted affect, hallucinations, delusions, etc., rarely occurs in prepuberal children. Mania, characterized by hyperactivity, euphoria, push of speech, and other symptoms characteristic of manic syndrome, likewise does occasionally present in prepuberal children. There is nothing to suggest that when these conditions do occur in a prepuberal child, the response to antipsychotics is any different from that in adults. These conditions occur more commonly in adolescence, and the indications there are more definitely established. Tourette's syndrome generally begins in childhood and is characterized by chronic motor and verbal tics. One psychotropic agent, haloperidol, has been the mainstay of therapeutic intervention with this disorder for quite a while. Its main problem from the standpoint of side effects in treating children with Tourette's syndrome is its tendency to produce cognitive dulling, which may affect academic performance in the classroom. For this reason, alternative drugs are being sought for the treatment of Tourette's syndrome, and clonidine recently has shown some promise (Cohen, et al., 1980).

There are three conditions that might be considered possible indications for the use of antipsychotics in childhood, these are: *pervasive developmental disorders,* certain symptoms of *mental retardation* and *attention deficit disorder with hyperactivity.* Considering the latter condition, the response of attention deficit disorder with hyperactivity to major tranquilizers such as the phenothiazines is considerably different from the response to stimulants. The major tranquilizers produce a decrease in activity level across all settings and may produce cognitive dulling. The change in activity level produced by stimulants seems to be fundamentally different, and cognitive function is improved, not impaired. Thus, the use of these drugs with this condition will occur only rarely. Some studies, such as that by Klein et al. (1980), suggest that a combination of methylphenidate and phenothiazine, such as thioridazine, may produce a somewhat better symptomatic improvement on an item-by-item basis, but not enough to be statistically significant compared to methylphenidate alone.

In the case of the use of the phenothiazines and other major tranquilizers with the pervasive developmental disorders, such as infantile autism, and with mental retardation, these drugs are not antipsychotic in the true sense of the word. What is being treated in these conditions is the secondary symptomatology, not the core symptomatology. Thus, such symptoms as hyperactivity and aggressiveness can be significantly improved in some children. The goal would be, of course, to help the children to be more amenable to other areas of therapeutic intervention, such as educational intervention, speech, and language training. These drugs will not produce the dramatic change in core symptomatology that one sees in adults with a true schizophrenic disorder.

Antimanic Drugs

The lithium ion was introduced as an effective drug for the active manic phase of manic depressive disease in adults. That remains its only definite indication in childhood. The review by Youngerman and Canino (1978) has shown that there are children in the prepuberal age range who present with a manic condition relatively indistinguishable from that seen in adults. Lithium has been found to produce as beneficial an effect in this condition in children and adolescents as in adults. In adults, lithium also seems to be effective in some cases of depression and seems to exert a prophylactic effect on the recurrence of both depressive and manic eposides. This kind of data is not yet available for children.

However, there are two possible indications for the use of lithium in children. Some data suggest that there are children who present with cyclical disorders, not necessarily classically manic and depressive in their clinical picture, who do get a positive response to lithium. Much of this data comes from the work of Annell (1969).

In adults there are some data to suggest that lithium may be effective in the treatment of aggressive behavior. This has been verified in children, especially in a number of studies with the mentally retarded, making this a possible indication for the use of lithium in childhood (Aman, in press).

Antianxiety Agents (Minor Tranquilizers)

As mentioned above, "minor tranquilizer" is a poor term for this class of compounds. "Antianxiety drugs" is a much better overall generic term. The ones most in use at present are the benzodiazepines. The outstanding indication for their use in *adults* is for the treatment of anticipatory anxiety. However, in children their use can only be considered a possible indication for the anxiety disorders of childhood, since there has been a relative lack of research of any type on the treatment of antianxiety disorders in childhood with any type of psychotropic agent.

The only definitely established indication for the use of antianxiety agents in childhood is *night terrors*. Valium apparently produces a significant improvement in night terrors. The mechanism is thought to be due to its inhibition of stage-four sleep.

SUMMARY AND CONCLUSIONS

This chapter has briefly attempted to review some of the general principles involved in the psychopharmacologic treatment of children and the major indications for the use of psychotropic drugs for specific psychiatric disorders. The interested reader is referred to very recent comprehensive reviews for a detailed discussion of the evidence to support the statements made in this chapter and for a discussion of the specific dosages and side effects of the medications discussed. Much more research needs to be done in two areas: (1) the long-term effectiveness of psychotropic drugs with many conditions in childhood, and (2) the use of psychotropic drugs alone compared to their use combined with other therapeutic modalities and compared to the other therapeutic modalities alone.

REFERENCES

Aman, M. Drugs, learning and the psychotherapies. In *Pediatric Psychopharmacology: The Use of Behavior Modifying Drugs in Children*, J. Werry, ed. Brunner/Mazel, New York (1978), pp. 79–108.
———. Psychoactive drugs in mental retardation. In *Treatment Issues and Innovations in Mental Retardation*, J.L. Matson and F. Andrasik, eds. Plenum Press, New York (in press).
American Psychiatric Association (APA). *Diagnostic and Statistical Manual of Mental Disorders (DSM-III)*. APA, Washington, D.C. (1980).
Annell, A. Lithium treatment of children and adolescents. *Acta Psychiatrica Scandinavica, 207*, 19–30 (1969).
Bradley, C. The behavior of children receiving benzedrine. *American Journal of Orthopsychiatry, 94*, 577–585 (1937).
Cantwell, D.P. *The Hyperactive Child—Diagnosis, Management, Current Research.* Spectrum, New York (1975).
———. CNS activating drugs in the treatment of hyperactive children. In *Controversy in Psychiatry*, J. Brady and H. Brodie, eds. W.B. Saunders, Philadelphia (1978).
Cantwell, D.P., and Carlson, G.A. Stimulants. In *Pediatric Psychopharmacology: The Use of Behavior Modifying Drugs in Children*, J. Werry, ed. Brunner/Mazel, New York (1978), pp. 171–207.
Cohen, D.J., Detlor, J., Young, J.G., and Shaywitz, B.A. Clonidine ameliorates Gilles de la Tourette syndrome. *Archives of General Psychiatry, 37*, 1350–1357 (1980).
Guy, W. *ECDEU Assessment Manual for Psychopharmacology*. National Institute of Mental Health, Psychopharmacology Research Branch, U.S. Department of Health, Education, and Welfare, Rockville, Md. (1976).
Hill, D. Amphetamine in psychopathic states. *British Journal of Addiction, 44*, 50–54 (1947).
Klein, D.F., Gittelman, R., Quitkin, R., and Rifkin, R. *Diagnosis and Drug Treatment of Psychiatric Disorders in Adults and Children*. Williams & Wilkins, Baltimore (1980).
Maletzky, B. d-Amphetamine and delinquency: Hyperkinesis persisting? *Diseases of the Nervous System, 35*, 543–547 (1974).
Quay, J. Classification. In *Psychopathological Disorders of Childhood*, 2nd ed., H. Quay and J. Werry, eds. Wiley, New York (1980).
Rutter, M., Graham, P., and Yule, W. A neuropsychiatric study in childhood. *Clinics in Developmental Medicine, Nos. 35/36*. Heinemann, London (1970).

Werry, J. *Pediatric Psychopharmacology: The Use of Behavior Modifying Drugs in Children.* Brunner/Mazel, New York (1978).
Youngerman, J., and Canino, I.A. Lithium carbonate use in children and adolescents. *Archives of General Psychiatry, 35,* 216–224 (1978).

BIBLIOGRAPHY

General

Anthony E.J., and Koupernik, C., eds. *The Child in His Family—The Impact of Disease and Death.* Wiley, New York (1973).
Azarnoff, P. Mediating the trauma of serious illness and hospitalization in childhood. *Children Today,* (1974).
Bergmann, T., and Freud, A. *Children in the Hospital.* International Universities Press, New York (1965).
Bowden, C.L., and Burstein, A.G. *Psychosocial Basis of Medical Practice: An Introduction to Human Behavior,* 2nd ed. Williams & Wilkins, Baltimore (1979).
Gellent, E. *Psychosocial Aspects of Pediatric Care.* Grune & Stratton, New York (1978).
Klinzing, D.R., and Klinzing, D.G. *The Hospitalized Child: Communication Techniques for Health Personnel.* Prentice-Hall, Englewood Cliffs, N.J. (1977).
Langford, W.S. Psychological aspects of pediatrics, physical illness and convalescence: Their meaning to the child. *Journal of Pediatrics, 33,* 242 (1948).
Melamed, B.G. Psychological preparation for hospitalization. In *Contribution to Medical Psychology,* Vol. 1, S. Rachman, ed. Pergamon Press (1977), pp. 43–74.
Minuchin, S., et al. A conceptual model of psychosomatic illness in children. *Archives of General Psychiatry, 32,* 1031 (1975).
Petrillo, M., and Sanger, S. *Emotional Care of Hospitalized Children: An Environmental Approach,* 2nd ed. J.B. Lippincott, Philadelphia (1980).
Prugh, D., and Eckhardt, L.O. Children's reactions to illness, hospitalization and surgery. In *Comprehensive Textbook of Psychiatry,* Vol. 2, A.M. Freedman, H.I. Kaplan, and B.J. Sakock, eds. Williams & Wilkins, Baltimore (1975), pp. 2100–2107.
Schowalter, J.E. Psychological reactions to physical illness and hospitalization in adolescence: A survey. *Journal of the American Academy of Child Psychiatry, 16,* 500–516 (1977).
Stocking, M., Rothney, W., Grosser, G., and Goodwin, R. Psychopathology in the pediatric hospital—implications for community health. *A.J.P.H.,* 551 (1972).

Preparation of Child for Hospitalization and/or Surgery

Hardgrove, C., Emotional innoculation: The 3 R's of preparation. *JACCH, 5,* 17 (1977).
Mellish, R.W.P. Preparation of a child for hospitalization and surgery. *Pediatric Clinics of North America, 16,* 543 (1969).

Psychological Considerations in Surgery

Blotcky, M.J., and Grossman, I. Psychological implications of childhood genito-urinary surgery. *Journal of the American Academy of Child Psychiatry,* *17,* 488 (1978).

Healy, M.H., and Hansen, H. Psychiatric management of limb amputation in a pre-school child. *Journal of the American Academy of Child Psychiatry,* *16,* 684-692 (1977).

Specific Topics in Pediatric Consultation-Liaison Psychiatry

Abuse

Green, A.H. Psychopathology of abused children. *Journal of the American Academy of Child Psychiatry, 17,* 92-103 (1978).

Green, A., Gaines, R.W., and Sandgrund, A. Child abuse: Pathological syndrome of family interaction. *American Journal of Psychiatry, 131,* 882 (1974).

Alopecia Areata

Mehlman, R.D., and Griesemer, R.D. Alopecia areata in the very young. *American Journal of Psychiatry, 125,* 605 (1968).

Asthma

Gauthier, Y., et al. The mother-child relationship and the development of auton-omy and self-assertion in young asthmatic children. *Journal of the American Academy of Child Psychiatry, 16,* 109-131 (1977).

Gauthier, Y., et al. Follow-up study of 35 asthmatic pre-school children. *Journal of the American Academy of Child Psychiatry, 17,* 679-694 (1978).

Bonding

Lozoff, B., Brittenham, G.M., Trause, M.A., Kennell, J.H., and Klaus, M.H. The mother-newborn relationship: Limits of adaptability. *Journal of Pediatrics, 91,* 1-12 (1977).

Cardiac Disorders

Gottesfeld, I.B. The family of the child with congenital heart disease. *Maternal Child Nursing,* 101-104 (1979).

Urzak, K. A child's cardiac catheterization—avoiding the potential risks. *Maternal Child Nursing,* 158-161 (1978).

Cerebral Palsy

Richardson, S.A. People with cerebral palsy talk for themselves. *Developmental Medicine and Child Neurology, 14,* 524-535 (1972).

Conversion Reactions

Rock, N.L. Conversion reactions in childhood: A clinical study on childhood neurosis. *Journal of the American Academy of Child Psychiatry, 10,* 65-93 (1971).

Cystic Fibrosis

Boyle, I.R., et al. Emotional adjustment of adolescents and young adults with cystic fibrosis. *Journal of Pediatrics, 88,* 318-326 (1976).

McCrae, W.M. Emotional problems in cystic fibrosis. *Physiotherapy, 61*, 252–254 (1975).

Tropauer, A., et al. Psychological aspects of the care of children with cystic fibrosis. *Amer. J. Dis. Child, 119*, 424–432 (1970).

Deafness
Galenson, E., et al. Assessment of development in the deaf child. *Journal of the American Academy of Child Psychiatry, 18*, 128–142 (1979).

Death
Green, M., and Solerit, A.J. Reaction to the threatened loss of a child: A vulnerable child syndrome. *Pediatrics, 58–66* (1964).

Jackson, P.L. The child's developing concept of death. *Nursing Forum, 14*, 204–215 (1975).

Encopresis
Levine, M.D. Children with encopresis: A descriptive analysis. *Pediatrics, 56*, 412–416 (1975).

Levine, M.D., and Bakow, H. Children with encopresis: A study of treatment outcome. *Pediatrics, 58*, 845–852 (1976).

Enuresis
Esman, A.H. Nocturnal enuresis. *Journal of the American Academy of Child Psychiatry, 16*, 150–158 (1977).

Hemophilia
Mattsson, A., and Gross, S. Social and behavioral studies on hemophiliac children and their families. *Journal of Pediatrics, 68*, 952–964 (1966).

Hysteria
Dubowitz, V., and Hersov, L. Management of children with non-organic (hysterical) disorders of motor function. *Developmental Medicine and Child Neurology, 18*, 358–368 (1976).

Incest
Rosenfeld, A.A., Nadelson, C.C., et al. Incest and sexual abuse of children. *Journal of the American Academy of Child Psychiatry, 16*, 327–339 (1977).

Leukemia
Heffron, W.A., et al. Group discussions with the parents of leukemic children. *Pediatrics, 52*, 831–840 (1973).

Refugees from Southeast Asia
Leyn, R.B. The challenge of caring for child refugees from S.E. Asia. *American Journal of Maternal Child Nursing*, 178–182 (1978).

Rumination
Flanagan, C.H. Rumination in infancy—past and present with a case report. *Journal of the American Academy of Child Psychiatry, 16*, 140–149 (1977).

Sleep Disturbance
Keith, P.R. Night terrors. *Journal of the American Academy of Child Psychiatry*, *14*, 477–489 (1975).

Spina Bifida
Dorner, S. Sexual interest and activity in adolescents with spina bifida. *Journal of Child Psychology and Psychiatry*, *18*, 229–237 (1977).

Stress
Jacobson, S.P. Stressful situations for neonatal ICU nurses. *American Journal of Maternal Child Nursing*, 144–150 (1978).

Trichotillomania (Foreign Body Ingestion)
Aleksandrowicz, M.K., and Mares, A.J. Trichotillomania and trichobezoar in an infant. *Journal of the American Academy of Child Psychiatry*, *17*, 533–539 (1978).

Ulcerative Colitis
McLean, G. An approach to the treatment of an adolescent with ulcerative colitis. *Canadian Psychiatric Association Journal*, *21*, 287–293 (1976).

2

Maternal Bonding and Infant Attachment

Charles W. Ralston and Mary J. O'Connor

The mother-child relationship has long been of concern to those who deal with the problems of children. Accompanying the recent awareness of the importance of early life to later development, there has been increased interest in the nature of the relationship that transpires between a mother and her newborn infant, and much research is being directed toward the identification of critical variables and the assessment of long-term effects of the process. The terms "bonding" and "attachment" have become a part of the daily vocabulary of professionals caring for infants and children. They receive increasing coverage in the lay press, and parents now frequently express concern about the consequences of obstetrical management on the relationship with their newborn. Parents also ask about how separations, as those occurring with preterm birth and later hospitalization, will influence their children emotionally. To be helpful when such questions are raised, child health professionals need a reasonable understanding of the concepts involved in bonding and attachment. In this chapter we hope to clarify the meaning of these terms and discuss some of the evidence that has aided our understanding of the processes.

Our discussion will be in terms of the relationship between mother and infant. This is because the mother generally has the primary role in infant care. However, this role is not restricted to the biological parent and when the term "mother" is used we imply the primary caregiver.

Bonding, as generally used, describes the unique, enduring emotional relationship that evolves in a mother toward her child. Although a mother's emotional tie to her infant is affected by many factors, both prenatal and postnatal, recent research has focused predominantly on events immediately following birth. Early and close contact between mother and newborn reportedly strengthens their relationship, and changes in their early interaction may be manifested in maternal behaviors later. Because of the focus on the early postnatal period, bonding is seen by some as a rapid process that occurs optimally in the minutes immediately following birth, when the mother is primed to receive her infant.

This view has led to the popular notion that the interaction immediately following delivery is critical to the long-term relationship between mother and child.

The term *attachment* is used frequently by clinicians to describe the relationship between mother and infant in both directions. Klaus and Kennell (1976), whose book helped popularize the term *bonding*, used it synonymously with *maternal attachment*. However, the more specific meaning of attachment refers to the infant's affectional tie to his mother, which begins to develop gradually over the first year of life. According to Bowlby's attachment theory (1969), this relationship is described in terms of a set of species-specific behaviors that act to attain or maintain proximity to the identified primary caregiver and, as such, are seen as behaviors that have preserved the species by keeping the vulnerable newborn near the protecting adult. The development of the infant's attachment seems to be dependent on the nature of the interaction with the mother. As bonding may be one of the important variables in determining this interaction, the two processes appear to be intimately related.

BONDING

The bonding process begins long before a child is born and continues after the delivery is complete. A woman's attitudes toward mothering reflect not only her own genetic endowment and her relationship with her own mother, but also socioeconomic status, cultural expectations, and the marital situation. Emotional support and experience with previous pregnancies are also important in preparing for the relationship. Bonding is already present at birth, as evidenced in the grieving seen in mothers whose infants die during or prior to delivery (Kennell, Slyter, and Klaus, 1970). In addition, the process continues long after delivery. Some parents report that the acceptance process continues for months and is influenced by the infant's own contribution to the interaction (Robson and Moss, 1970).

Recent research on bonding has focused on the interaction between mother and infant in the immediate postnatal period. There have been a number of reasons for this orientation. Observations of several animal species indicate that there is a critical period immediately following birth in which specific behaviors must occur if normal mothering is to follow (Rhinegold, 1963). Though there is no evidence for a similar critical period in humans, there is a belief that the mother, immediately postpartum, may be especially sensitive to contact with her newborn. It is hypothesized that during this period she forms a strong affectional bond more easily than she will at any later time. The concept of the "sensitive period" is further supported by the infant's period of extreme alertness following delivery, which seems particularly suited to capture the mother at a time when she seeks confirmation of her prenatal expectations. A second reason for focusing on the postnatal period has been the concern that modern medical management of the birth process has separated newborn infant and family in a way not often seen in human history. This has been in the face of a growing body of information showing that separation is not necessarily indicated for disease prevention. Finally, early retrospective studies of "mothering disorders," like child abuse and nonorganic failure to thrive, seem to show an overrepresentation of mothers who delivered prior to term. If preterm birth, a natural experiment in separation, produces such difficulties, the separation accompanying a routine birth might also disrupt the normal bonding process and make mothering more difficult.

The Klaus and Kennell (1976) study of 28 disadvantaged, predominantly single mothers has been widely reported in support of the existence of a maternal sensitive period immediately following birth. The authors have argued effectively that modern hospital procedures separate infant and mother unnecessarily and that the separation may have long-term consequences. Their study design allowed 14 mothers to have one hour of skin-to-skin contact with their newborns after delivery and five extra hours of contact a day for the next three days. The control group received "traditional" management, including a glimpse of the newborn at birth and brief contacts for feeding beginning at 6–12 hours of age. When questioned one month after delivery, the extra-contact mothers responded that they were more likely to attend to their crying infants and felt more uncomfortable leaving them with someone else. They were observed to stand closer to their children during a physical exam and to soothe more often when the children cried. Of 25 behaviors assessed during a feeding, they showed more *en face* looking and more fondling (Klaus et al., 1972).

When seen after one year, the extra-contact mothers again soothed their infants and assisted in the physical exam more than did the controls. Of the mothers who returned to work, the controls were less likely to miss their infants. However, several other important comparisons, including response to separation, developmental assessment, and interaction during free play, did not yield meaningful differences between extra contact and control groups (Kennell et al., 1974). A language assessment of give randomly selected mother-infant pairs from each group at two years found the extra-contact mothers communicating in a way that was more complex and more contingent on the child's responses. These mothers used more questions, fewer commands, and more words per proposition (Ringler et al., 1975). The same contact children at five years showed comprehension of significantly more complex phrases (Klaus and Kennell, 1976). The authors concluded that these studies are evidence that relatively minor alterations in early contact may have significant long-term effects.

Though this research has been instrumental in helping to bring about changes in hospital policies that separate mothers from their newborns, there has been concern that the findings might lack generalizability because the population studied was limited in number and in social-class composition. Few studies reported to date have used a similar early and extended contact design. One such report in an American disadvantaged population (Siegel et al., 1980) partially replicated the findings of Klaus and Kennell in that contact seemed to significantly facilitate the mother's acceptance of her infant and increased her likelihood of consoling the infant when crying. Although the study provided support for the influence of early contact, it also indicated that contact is less important than other influences, such as maternal background (as defined by race, age, marital status, education, and I.Q.).

While the studies cited above assessed mother-infant bonding following several manipulations in hospital routine, other studies have attempted to demonstrate the importance of specific manipulations on the bonding process. Hales and associates (Hales et al., 1977), investigating the significance of the timing of extra contact, allowed one group of Guatemalan mothers 45 minutes of skin contact immediately following delivery. A second group had the same 45-minute contact but at 12 hours of age. At 36 hours, the early-contact group showed more "affectionate behavior," but the difference was determined entirely by one variable—en face looking. Though this finding is reported as evidence for the importance of timing of contact, it should be noted that the early-contact mothers had known their infants for 12 hours longer at 36 hours of age. This difference, rather than the time of contact, may have been the more important variable.

De Chateau (1979) has recently reviewed his experience with a population of middle-class Swedish mothers, in which the effect of 15–20 minutes of skin-to-skin contact following delivery was explored. Management was the same as in the controls after the first 30 minutes. Observed 36 hours after birth, primiparous mothers experiencing early contact displayed behavior more similar to that of experienced mothers than to first-time mothers with no early contact. However, of the 35 behaviors assessed, only three were significantly different with respect to the contact variable, and only one of these—amount of holding—seems logically related to bonding. The mother-infant pairs were assessed at three months, and again differences based on the contact variable were found. This time, of 61 behaviors, extra-contact mothers showed more en face looking and kissing and less cleaning of their infants. Significantly more extra-contact mothers were breast feeding at three months, and they reported fewer problems with night feedings. The partial follow-up at one year revealed more advanced development in the contact infants and more physical contact and talking in their interactions. The findings of the study must be qualified by the observation that most differences were determined by mothers of male infants. The author states that he does not believe that the early contact alone explains the differences, but, rather, the early exchange of signals may be a way of getting the relationship off on the right foot so that later mother-infant synchronization may proceed more smoothly (de Chateau, 1979).

Behavioral differences at two and four days have been reported in a similar Swedish population in which mothers received five minutes or one hour of early postnatal contact (Carlsson et al., 1978). The prolonged early-contact mothers displayed more behaviors requiring contact with their infants. By six weeks, however, their behaviors were equivalent in a feeding sequence, and the mothers were not systematically different in their feelings about the management of the pregnancy or their plans for mothering (Carlsson et al., 1979). Similarly, Taylor and associates (Campbell and Taylor, 1979), in a study of middle-class American women experiencing one hour of early contact at 30 minutes of age, found no detectable differences in mother-infant interaction during feeding or in the maternal perceptions of her infant up to one month of age, as compared to controls without such contact.

Thus, evidence for a positive influence of early postnatal contact alone on maternal-infant interaction has been equivocal. Measurable differences have not been large, and they have tended to disappear early in infancy. This has led some researchers to look for other possible influences in the neonatal period.

One such approach has been to focus on the effect of prolonged exposure of mother and infant during the hospital stay by studying mothers who room-in. Ideally, rooming-in mothers begin to assume responsibility for the infant's care in a setting where they can ask questions and get help from experienced professionals. Later, these mothers should be more relaxed and competent in their caretaking roles. If the new mother's early interaction with her infant is more comfortable, later interaction may be smoother and there may be fewer problems of parenting. These ideas are supported in a recent study comparing indigent mothers randomly assigned to rooming-in or to traditional postnatal management groups (O'Connor et al., 1980). When the charts of 301 children were reviewed at an average of 17 months, serious parenting difficulties were seen in 1.5 percent of the rooming-in families and in seven percent of the controls. The authors concluded that this extended exposure, even without early contact, was helpful in preventing later parenting deficiencies by allowing greater opportunity for mother and infant to adapt to each other. More synchronous adaptation in the first few days may lead to greater skill and confidence in the later mother-infant interaction and thus decrease the chance for problems.

A related and important issue deals with the concern that the prolonged separation that families of preterm infants experience makes difficult the occurrence of the normal bonding process. It is reasoned that incomplete bonding may produce an abnormal parent-child relationship and lead to disturbances in parenting (such as battered-child syndrome or nonorganic failure to thrive). Furthermore, when visiting patterns of mothers to the preterm nursery were examined, a correlation between disorders of mothering and infrequent visitation was found (Fanaroff et al., 1972). The interpretation of this line of thought has been questioned because of the difficulty of separating the added effects of social class, financial and emotional stress of hospitalization on the family, and the increased likelihood that the preterm infant will have significant, ongoing medical problems.

Some researchers have found it valuable to investigate variables other than separation that might mediate the association between preterm birth and parenting disorders. A recent study of infants weighing less than 1500 grams at birth (Boyle, Griffen, and Fitzhardinge, 1977) found no evidence that preterm birth itself had a significant negative effect on the parental attitudes three to five years later. Rather, their attitudes were related to persiting neurological and intellectual difficulties. Minde and his colleagues in Toronto have made careful observations of the behaviors and visiting patterns of parents to the newborn Intensive Care Unit (ICU) (Minde et al., 1978). Some mothers consistently seemed to interact more than others, and this difference persisted up to three months following discharge. The more interactive mothers also visited and phoned more. The extent of the child's illness was not a determinant of the interaction. From a psychiatric interview, it appeared that, while the more interactive mothers came from intact families with ample social supports, the least interactive tended to lack the support of their spouses and had few friends. Similarly, Collingswood and Alberman (1979) found that only a small subgroup of mothers of preterm infants showed signs of conflict in the mother-child relationship five years after delivery. These mothers were younger at the birth of the child, were less prepared for pregnancy, and had worse relationships with their own parents.

Finally, Leiderman (1978) has reviewed the large prospective study, conducted at Stanford, on the effect of early parental contact with the preterm infant. In this study, mothers who were allowed physical contact with their preterm infants from the second or third day of life, and caretaking responsibilities whenever possible, were compared with mothers having only visual contact for the first 3 to 12 weeks. No significant differences were found in maternal behavior with the infants up to 21 months following discharge. By 21 months, socioeconomic status, sex, and birth order were far more potent predictors of maternal activity than were conditions surrounding birth. Nevertheless, there was evidence that the preterm birth placed a strain on the family that could be modified by physical contact. The families that were allowed only minimal contact accounted for the only two relinquishments and five of the seven divorces occurring in the first 21 months. It was the author's feeling that the evidence supported a stressing effect on family dynamics rather than on mother-infant interaction.

One important variable, not often considered, concerns the infant's contribution to the bonding process. An understanding of this contribution may be especially necessary when dealing with the preterm or defective newborn. The mother of such a child is presented with a baby that does not conform to her preconceived ideal infant. Such an infant may evoke anxious or even aversive feelings in the mother. There is evidence that some preterm infants may be more difficult to arouse and less responsive than the full-term infant and that these differences may persist for some time (Parmelee et al., 1980). Field (1977) describes the interaction of preterm, postmature, and the full-term mother-infant dyads. At 3½ months, the preterm and postmature infants showed significantly less gazing during maternal activity than did the full terms. However, only the preterms were separated in the neonatal period, suggesting that factors other than separation may be active in producing the differences. Since the less interactive infants seemed to be that way also in the newborn period, the crucial factor may be a difference in interactive styles that persists at least through the first few months.

It is postulated that because of interactive limitations, it may be more difficult for some preterm or congenitally defective infants to inspire a feeling of competence in their mothers. This lack of reinforcement may make the bonding process more difficult. It must be remembered, however, that most parents in these situations do form healthy, positive relationships with their children. Diminished responsiveness on the infant's part does not necessarily mean that the mothers are any less interactive. In fact, some mothers seem to respond to the challenge of the difficult child with even more effort and in doing so may compensate for some deficits on the child's part (Parmelee et al., 1980). Though the birth of a preterm or defective infant may represent a stress to the formation of the normal emotional tie, this does not mean that the bonding process will not take place or that the bond will not be as strong as it is in other situations.

Thus, it seems clear that factors other than postdelivery management have important effects on the evolving mother-child relationship. The literature cited here, though not exhaustive, is representative of the work in the field to date. While early and extended contact between the mother and her newborn is a natural and usually pleasurable experience, the evidence does not support its having a major impact on the process of bonding. This is not to say there is no effect. For the mother at risk for interactional difficulties, even a small positive influence may be enough to boost her over the hypothetical threshold for parenting adequacy.

The "sensitive period" concept implies that this early contact acts to establish the mother's instinctual emotional bond to the infant more easily than is possible at any other time. A different interpretation, which is perhaps more in keeping with the idea of man as an adaptive, dynamic creature, would view early contact as an opportunity for the mother to better understand her new child. The alertness and responsibility of the newborn in the minutes following delivery may serve not only to reassure her of his well-being, but also encourage a general interest in his behavior that persists throughout the hospitalization. Increased exposure provides a chance for her to become familiar with the baby's response patterns prior to having to assume total responsibility for the care at home.

Knowing what to expect may lead to more comfort and competence in the care-giving role. In a supportive hospital environment, the inexperienced mother may learn coping strategies for problems as they arise. If this makes the mother-infant interaction in the first months smoother, strengthening of the later relationship might logically be expected.

Professionals dealing with mothers and infants should be aware of two poten-tial problems that have accompanied the focus on postnatal management and the use of the "sensitive period" concept. The first has been the tendency to view changes in postnatal management as a panacea for all problems of maternal-child interaction. If, as we have seen, problems of parenting have their origin in many diverse factors, both pre- and postnatal, it would seem likely that an intervention aimed at only a part of the bonding process would meet with limited success. The second major concern is that mothers who are unable to experience early contact may feel that the ensuing relationship cannot be completely normal. Hence, the mother with obstetrical complications or the mother of a preterm or adopted infant may worry unnecessarily about what she has missed. It is impor-tant for these mothers to know that the early contact, so often talked about, is not a requisite for a strong mother-infant relationship.

ATTACHMENT

In addition to concern about the impact of medical intervention on the early bond of the mother to the infant, health care professionals have begun to examine the impact of later interventions, such as hospitalization, on the devel-opment of the attachment of infant to mother. A description of the attachment process may help to make professionals aware of problems that may arise in a medical setting and suggest ways in which to intervene.

The attachment theory of Bowlby (1969) has its origins in several important trends in the behavioral sciences, including psychoanalytic theory, ethology, neurophysiology, and the cognitive psychology of Piaget. The major assumption of attachment theory is that attachment behaviors exhibited by the human infant are part of a species-specific behavioral system that operates to promote and maintain proximity to a primary caretaker, thus ensuring protection of the infant from danger. This behavioral system has developed through the process of evolution in order to ensure the survival of the species. Far from being a purely instinctual theory, Bowlby's attachment theory states that the constitu-tional predisposition of the infant present at birth becomes modified and elabor-ated through experience with the environment—particularly through social inter-action with the primary caretaker.

The specific types of behaviors comprising the behavioral attachment system of the infant can be grouped into two main classes: signaling behaviors and approach behaviors. Signaling behaviors serve to attract and keep the caregiver close and include crying, smiling, babbling, calling, and gesturing. Approach behaviors bring the child to the mother and allow for maintaining proximity. These include sucking, clinging, crawling, and walking. All of the behaviors classified as part of the attachment system can serve other behavioral systems. It is only under certain situations, when the behaviors serve to promote and maintain proximity to the mother, that they are operating in the service of the attachment system. For example, smiling at another child constitutes social behavior that is not serving an attachment function. Although it is common practice to speak of the mother's attachment to her infant, Bowlby reserves the term *attachment behavior* exclusively for the behavior exhibited by the infant toward the attachment figure. The behavior of the parent that is reciprocal to the attachment behavior of the infant is termed *caretaking behavior*.

In general, conditions that produce high states of arousal in the infant also activate the attachment behavioral system. Among the internal variables that may lead to activation are hunger, pain, cold, or illness. External environmental variables include the departure or absence of an attachment figure, lack of response or rejection from such a figure, and unfamiliar situations or individuals.

The nature of the child's relationship to the mother to a large extent determines the attachment behavior exhibited toward her. Stress, such as that elicited by the presence of a strange adult, leads the infant to seek contact with the attachment figure. If the infant is secure with the mother, contact with her is comforting, and her mere presence allows the infant to explore the novel stranger. A child who is chronically anxious about the mother's accessibility and responsiveness will show greater fear of strangers than one who is securely attached, and will not be able to leave the mother to explore.

As Bowlby describes it, attachment to the mother figure develops gradually during the first year of life. In the initial phase of development, shortly after birth, attachment behaviors are simply structured, almost reflexive in nature, and are readily elicited by stimuli provided by adult caretakers. Research has shown that infants are programmed to respond in specific ways to stimuli that are characteristic of human beings. For example, infants respond more strongly to sounds that are within the fundamental frequencies of the human voice (Eisenberg, 1965) and to visual stimuli that have the characteristics of the human face (Haith, Bergman, and Moore, 1977).

During the first phase of the development of attachment, the baby is interested and responsive to all people. His behavior includes orientation to and gazing at people, tracking movements of the eyes, primitive grasping and reaching, smiling, and cessation of crying in response to the human voice or face. In addition, the infant can actively seek or maintain contact with caregivers by sucking and molding when held. Bowlby has suggested that these primitive behaviors become organized by a process of learning through interaction with the environment. According to Ainsworth, during this first phase of development the infant begins to build up expectations of how the human environment will respond (Ainsworth et al., 1978). This phase terminates when the infant is capable of making discriminations among people, in particular in discriminating the mother from others, which usually occurs at around 8 to 12 weeks of age.

The second phase lasts about six months and is characterized by the infant's ability to discriminate among people. The infant begins to direct attachment behaviors more toward one figure, and this figure, usually the mother, is generally more successful than others in terminating attachment behavior such as crying. The baby's repertoire of attachment behaviors expands to include coordinated reaching. He knows the specific features of the primary caretaker, but his attachment to that caretaker is not fully developed.

The third phase, that of "clear-cut attachment" (Ainsworth et al., 1978), occurs sometime during the second half of the first year of life and continues through the second and third years. Rather than relying heavily on signaling behavior to bring the mother to him, the child now actively approaches the mother and stays with her by means of locomotion. His discrimination of the attachment figure increases and his repertoire of responses extends to include following the mother, greeting her, and using her as a secure base from which to explore. Other behaviors in the service of the attachment behavior system emerge, including holding on to the mother and using language to call her. Concurrently during this phase, friendly and indiscriminate responses to unfamiliar people decrease and are replaced by behaviors characteristic of wariness or fear.

During the fourth phase in the development of attachment, the mother is understood as an independent object who comes and goes and who is persistent in time and space. The essential feature of this phase is the lessening of egocentricity in the child to the point that the child is capable of seeing things from his mother's point of view and thus is able to infer feelings and motives, goals, and plans that might influence her behavior. To the extent that the child has developed a representational model of his mother to include inferences of this sort, he is able to accommodate his behavior to her plans. Bowlby states that when phase four is reached, the mother and child develop a relationship which he terms a "partnership." This phase occurs in most children around the third year. Although Bowlby was specifically concerned with the attachment of a child to the mother figure, the processes implicit in phase four were conceived as continuing throughout life and as being characteristic of mature attachments, which include figures other than the mother.

Research on attachment of the child to the mother was pioneered by Ainsworth and her co-workers, using the strange-situation procedure, a standardized method for exploring attachment behavior in one-year-olds. Since Ainsworth's original work, knowledge of the attachment process has expanded considerably, and most studies agree that there is a high congruence between the quality of mother-infant interaction and the quality of the child's attachments. Mothers of securely attached infants are more sensitively responsive to their infant's signals and communications and are more reciprocal and contingent in their interactions (Ainsworth and Bell, 1970; Bell and Ainsworth, 1972; Blehar, Lieberman, and Ainsworth, 1977). Furthermore, infants who know that their needs will be met and their signals responded to develop certain expectations about their environment as well as feelings of mastery and competence (Stayton, Hogan, and Ainsworth, 1971; Lewis et al., 1969; White, 1959). This conclusion is supported by a study by Matas, Ahrend, and Sroufe (1978), who examined the relation between the quality of infant attachment, mother's behavior, and two-year infant competence in various areas of functioning. Based upon the assumption that a well-functioning or competent infant is one who has formed an attachment relationship that supports active exploration and mastery of the environment, Matas et al. hypothesized that securely attached infants would later exhibit more autonomous functioning in the area of affective development and problem-solving style. According to the quality of their attachment relationship at 18 months, 48 infants were classified as secure, ambivalent, or avoidant in their attachments. On two-year assessments, infants classified as securely attached showed significantly more symbolic play and were more enthusiastic, positive, and persistent in the problem-solving task. Infants classified as avoidant or ambivalent in their attachment relationships showed poorer-quality adaptation at two years. The infants did not differ in cognitive functioning, as measured by the Bayley examination. Although the infant attachment behaviors at 18 months were presumed to reflect the quality of the infant's attachment to the mother, they also were presumed to reflect maternal sensitivity to infant signals and the quality of the mother-infant interaction. This hypothesis was confirmed in that mothers of securely attached infants performed more competently, as measured by their supportive presence and quality of assistance to the infant, than those of infants in other groups.

The finding of short-term association between early attachment and later social, emotional, and cognitive development has caused concern among health care professionals, who are aware that frequent and/or prolonged hospitalization of an infant may impact on the mother-infant relationship and, consequently, on the attachment process itself. Hospitalization can influence attachment in one of two ways: it can disrupt an ongoing attachment process or, in younger infants, it can cause it never to develop.

The response of the infant to a disruption in the attachment process following separation from the primary caretaker has been most clearly demonstrated by Robertson in his description of the behavior of children 15 to 30 months of age staying for a limited time in residential nurseries or hospital wards (Robertson, 1970). Infants in this situation show a predictable sequence of behavior consisting of protest, despair, and, finally, detachment. During the protest period, the child appears acutely distressed at the loss of the caretaker. He cries loudly, thrashes about, and continually searches for the mother, rejecting all alternative figures. During the period of despair the infant is still preoccupied with the missing mother, but his active physical movements decrease in intensity and frequency. The child makes few demands on the substitute caregiver, is quiet, and appears in a state of mourning. The onset of the detachment period is often viewed by professional staff as an indication that the infant has recovered from his withdrawal during the despair stage. The infant no longer rejects other caretakers, smiles, and is even sociable. When the mother visits, however, the infant may ignore her, turn away, and treat her like a stranger. If the stay is long, the infant may become attached to members of the nursing staff; but as more and more people are involved in his care, he may attach less and less to succeeding figures and, in time, may not attach at all. His behavior, however, may appear cheerful and adaptive to his unusual environment, although socially superficial.

Some investigators have suggested that the patterns described above may not be present in all infants and that variables other than separation might account for variability in response patterns. These variables include the nature of the strange environment itself, pain or illness associated with the hospital, the age of the child at hospitalization, the relationship between the child and mother, and the length of separation. In one study, Branstetter (1969) was able to demonstrate that the provision of a single mother substitute reduced the intensity of the reaction to hospitalization. In this study, the infant showed attachment to the substitute caregiver, although the mother remained the primary attachment figure.

In contrast to studies involving a disruption in the ongoing process of attachment, perhaps the clearest examples of failure for normal attachment to develop are found in the studies of infants separated from their mothers shortly after birth and raised in institutions. The most systematic research in this area has been conducted by Provence and Lipton (1962), who studied 75 infants who were institutionalized at less than three weeks of age. These infants were then compared with a group of home-reared infants. The effects of institutionalization on development were seen as early as at three months. The babies vocalized less, were late to discriminate between face and mask and between different individuals, made fewer social overtures, showed restricted expressive movements, and no attachment (at 12 months) to any particular person. On follow-up at 18 months, after the infants had been returned to a normal home situation, there were residual impairments of mild to severe degree in the area of "emotional relationships, in aspects of control and modulation of impulse, and in areas of thinking and learning that reflect multiple adaptive and defensive capacities and the development of flexibility in thought and action" (Provence and Lipton, 1962, p. 158).

Our studies of infants chronically hospitalized at UCLA Medical Center for several months following birth replicate many of the findings of Provence and Lipton. Most striking was that the infants we studied had problems in social interaction and in the development of attachment behaviors. At around four months, these infants were not discriminating in their responses to the mother, as opposed to a stranger, and were less sensitive to the subtle cues involved in eliciting and maintaining interaction with an adult. In the terminology of attachment theorists, hospitalized infants were slow to reach the second phase of development, during which the infant begins to direct attachment behaviors more toward one figure than to others. Mothers of these infants would often comment, "He doesn't know that I'm his mother." They often expressed concern that their infants were more responsive to their nurse caretakers than to them.

At around eight months, the hospitalized babies would try to elicit social interaction with a stranger, showing few signs of wariness. In contrast, a wariness of strange people in normal infants begins to appear as early as the fourth month of life and becomes increasingly apparent between the ages of 8 and 12 months (Bronson, 1972). Although fear/wariness of strangers was late to develop in hospitalized infants, once it did develop—usually after the infant had returned home—it was extreme, indicating high arousal with exaggeration of attachment behaviors in the presence of the mother.

There has been much discussion concerning what it is about the institutional or hospital environment that is responsible for the retarding effects on the child. Casler (1961) has argued effectively that it is not separation from the mother figure per se that is detrimental to normal growth and development but the environmental deprivation suffered by infants in nonstimulating institutions. Bowlby and Ainsworth have suggested that in the early months the mother figure *is* the main source of stimulation for the infant, and in the mother-infant interaction the infant is allowed the greatest opportunity for exploration of the larger environment.

An important theoretical approach to understanding the mother-infant relationship and its impact upon the child's attachment and, indeed, on the child's overall social and cognitive development, has been articulated in theories of social competence (Goldberg, 1977; Lewis et al., 1969; White, 1959). Social competence models argue that the infant is instrumental in establishing social conditions supportive of development and that the social relations of both infant and caregiver are mediated by mutual enhancement of "feelings of efficacy" (White, 1959). Conditions that contribute to feelings of efficacy depend upon the extent to which both caregiver and infant provide each other with contingent experiences. In order for normal attachment to proceed, interaction between caregiver and infant must be perceived as contingent; that is, each must presume the behavior of the other is a response to his own behavior (Ainsworth and Bell, 1974; Goldberg, 1977; Lewis and Goldberg, 1969).

The more mother and infant experience one another in these contingent interactions, the more elaborated and established these responses become. For example, the baby's auditory attention is encouraged and augmented by a process of feedback and learning by both mother and infant in the dyad. The infant's interest in the mother's voice is likely to lead the mother to talk to him more, which, in turn, causes the infant to pay attention and respond to the sounds she makes. Thus, the vocal and auditory interaction between the mother-infant pair increases. As has been demonstrated by Stern (1977) in his analysis of mother-infant interaction, there is a clear and integrated pattern of mutual and reciprocal interaction which has its basis in consistent inborn patterns of behavior that the baby exhibits from birth and to which the mother responds in a very stereotypic manner. The behavior of both partners changes in the trans-action, within certain limits, as a function of learning and mutual interaction (Sameroff and Chandler, 1975).

The appropriateness of the caregiver's interaction with the infant will deter-mine, to a large extent, much of the infant's early conceptualization of the envi-ronment. In addition, the consistency of the caregiver's interaction with the infant will provide opportunities for the development of expectancies in appro-priate social interaction and will form a basis for feelings of love, trust, and security.

Our observations have indicated that the long-term hospitalization of an infant results in situations that may interfere with mother-infant interaction and feelings of competency. One can only speculate about the specific nature of the influence of hospitalization on the mother and the infant; however, mutual responsiveness, upon which expectancies are built and feelings of competence achieved, is difficult to maintain during hospitalization. The mother's awareness of the infant's temporal routine and interactive cues is impaired under these unusual circumstances. She must relinquish most of the infant's care to nurses and doctors. Stress placed on her as a consequence of the hospitalization of a child, and possible guilt associated with it, can only serve to further disrupt the interaction. In addition to diminishing the mother's own feelings of competence, the workings of the hospital itself may result in disorganization in the infant's development.

CONCLUSION

In this chapter we have attempted to define bonding and attachment and have discussed research supporting the importance of these processes for the mother-child relationship. We have described how this relationship normally evolves and some of the ways by which it may be disrupted. It has been useful to conceptualize bonding as an affectional relationship of the mother to the infant, initiated prenatally and strengthened throughout life. Attachment has been viewed as an infant's emotional tie to the mother and is presumed to be manifested in attachment behaviors that the infant initiates toward her. The mother-infant interaction acts to establish and maintain both bonding and attachment.

Perhaps the most remarkable feature of the bonding and attachment processes is that most mothers and infants, regardless of the obstacles encountered, form healthy positive ties to each other. However, interactional problems do arise, and there is much concern about how they might be minimized or avoided. Because such difficulties have their origins in the diverse medical, social, and emotional factors of the individual family, an intervention program should be broadly focused and not limited to a single aspect of either process. A comprehensive support program might reasonably provide prenatal education and psychological help when necessary. The management of the birth process could offer, in addition to early infant contact, a mother- and family-oriented approach, allowing time for adaptation to the new infant. Mobilization of available support services and the provision of sensitive, developmentally oriented pediatric care could facilitate a more relaxed relationship between mother and child and help avoid later interactional difficulties. Helping the family cope with perceived and real stressors may allow the mother more opportunity for appropriate and responsive interaction with her infant, thus leading to more secure infant attachment and healthier development. If the young child requires hospitalization, the mother should be allowed the opportunity for normal interaction when possible. Intervention in several areas of family functioning, such as providing care for siblings, offering counseling for the parents, and involving appropriate community support agencies, may be most helpful. An approach with this orientation will not "immunize" a family against emotional or parenting problems, but does offer the opportunity to better understand the stressors that act to disrupt the family's functioning. By knowing each family better, our supportive interventions might address more specifically the family's basic needs.

REFERENCES

Ainsworth, M.D.S., and Bell, S.M.V. Attachment, exploration, and separation illustrated by the behavior of one-year-olds in a strange situation. *Child Development, 41,* 49–67 (1970).

–––. Mother-infant interaction and the development of competence. In *The Growth of Competence,* K.G. Connolly and J. Bruner, eds. Academic Press, New York (1974).

Ainsworth, M.D.S., Blehar, M.C., Waters, E., and Wall, S. *Patterns of Attachment.* Lawrence Erlbaum Associates, New York (1978).

Bell, S.M., and Ainsworth, M.D.S. Infant crying and maternal responsiveness. *Child Development, 43*, 1171-1190 (1972).

Bibring, G.L., Dwyer, T.F., Huntington, D.S., and Valenstein, A.F. A study of the psychological processes in pregnancy of the earliest mother-child relationship. I. Some propositions and comments. *Psychoanalytic Study of the Child, 16*, 9-27 (1961).

Blehar, M.C., Lieberman, A.F., and Ainsworth, M.D.S. Early face-to-face interaction and its relation to later infant-mother attachment. *Child Development, 48*, 182-194 (1977).

Bowlby, J. *Attachment and Loss: Attachment (Vol I)*. Basic Books, New York (1969).

Boyle, M., Griffen, A., and Fitzhardinge, P. The very low birthweight infant: Impact on parents during the preschool years. *Early Human Development, 1*, 191-201 (1977).

Branstetter, E. The young child's response to hospitalization: Separation and anxiety or lack of mother care. *American Journal of Public Health, 59*, 92-97 (1969).

Bronson, G.W. Infants' reactions to unfamiliar persons and novel objects. *Monographs of the Society for Research in Child Development 37* (1972).

Campbell, S.B., and Taylor, P.M. Bonding and attachment: Theoretical issues. *Seminars in Perinatology, 3*, 3-13 (1979).

Carlsson, F.G., Fagerberg, H., Horneman, G., Hwang, C., Larsson, K., Rodholm, M., Schaller, J., Danielsson, B., and Cundewall, C. Effects of amount of contact between mother and child on the mother's nursing behavior. *Developmental Psychobiology, 11*, 143-150 (1978).

―――. Effects of various amounts of contact between mother and child on the mother's nursing behavior: A follow-up study. *Infant Behavior and Development, 2*, 209-214 (1979).

Casler, L. Maternal deprivation: A critical review of the literature. *Monographs of the Society for Research in Child Development, 26* (1961).

Collingswood, J., and Alberman, A. Separation at birth and the mother-child relationship. *Developmental Medicine and Child Neurology, 21*, 608-618 (1979).

De Chateau, P. Effects of hospital practices on synchrony in the development of the infant-parent relationship. *Seminars in Perinatology, 3*, 45-60 (1979).

Eisenberg, R.B. Auditory behavior in the human neonate. *Journal of Auditory Research, 5*, 159-177 (1965).

Fanaroff, A.A., Kennell, J.H., and Klaus, M.H. Follow-up of low birthweight infants—the predictive value of maternal visiting patterns. *Pediatrics, 49*, 288-290 (1972).

Field, T.M. Effects of early separation, interactive deficits, and experimenter manipulations on infant-mother face-to-face interaction. *Child Development, 48*, 763-771 (1977).

Goldberg, S. Social competence in infancy: A model of parent-infant interaction. *Merrill Palmer Quarterly, 23*, 163-177 (1977).

Haith, M.M., Bergman, T., and Moore, M.J. Eye contact and face scanning in early infancy. *Science, 198*, 853-855 (1977).

Hales, D.J., Lozoff, B., Sosa, R., and Kennell, J.H. Defining the limits of the maternal sensitive period. *Developmental Medicine and Child Neurology, 19*, 454-461 (1977).

Kennell, J.H., Jerauld, R., Wolfe, H., Chester, D., Kreger, N.C., Mc Alpine, W., Steffa, M., and Klaus, M.H. Maternal behavior one year after early and extended post-partum contact. *Developmental Medicine and Child Neurology, 16,* 172–179 (1974).

Kennell, J.H., Slyter, H., and Klaus, M.H. The mourning response of parents to the death of a newborn infant. *New England Journal of Medicine, 283,* 344–349 (1970).

Klaus, M.H., Jerauld, R., Kreger, N., Mc Alpine, W., Steffa, M., and Kennel, J.H. Maternal attachment: The importance of the first post-partum days. *New England Journal of Medicine, 286,* 460–463 (1972).

Klaus, M.H., and Kennell, J.H. *Maternal-Infant Bonding.* C.V. Mosby, St. Louis (1976).

Leiderman, P.H. The critical period hypothesis revisited: Mother to infant social bonding in the neonatal period. In *Early Developmental Hazards: Predictions and Precautions,* F.D. Horowitz, ed. Westview Press, Boulder, Colo. (1978), pp. 43–77.

Lewis, M., Goldberg, S., and Campbell H. A developmental study of information processing within the first three years of life: response decrement to a redundant signal. *Monographs of the Society for Research in Child Development, 34* (1969).

Matas, L., Arend, R.A., and Sroufe, L.A. Continuity of adaptation in the second year: The relationship between quality of attachment and later competence. *Child Development, 49,* 547–556 (1978).

Minde, K., Trehub, S., Corter, C., Boukydis, C., Gelhoffer, L., and Marton, P. Mother-child relationships in the premature nursery: An observational study. *Pediatrics, 61,* 373–379 (1978).

O'Connor, S., Vietze, P., Sherrod, K.B., Sandler, H.M., and Altemeier, W.A. Reduced incidence of parenting inadequacy following rooming-in. *Pediatrics, 66,* 176–182 (1980).

Parmelee, A.H., Beckwith, L., Cohen, S.E., and Sigman, M. Social influences on infants at medical risk for behavioral difficulties. Presented at the First World Congress on Infant Psychiatry, Estoril, Portugal (April, 1980).

Provence, S., and Lipton, R.C. *Infants in Institutions.* International Universities Press, New York (1962).

Rhinegold, H.R., ed. *Maternal Behavior in Mammals.* Wiley, New York (1963).

Ringler, N.M., Kennell, J.H., Jarvella, R., Navojosky, B.J., and Klaus, M.H. Mother-to-child speech at 2 years—effects of early postnatal contact. *Journal of Pediatrics, 86,* 141–144 (1975).

Robertson, J. *Young Children in Hospitals.* Tavistock, London (1970).

Robson, K.S., and Moss, H.A. Patterns and determinants of maternal attachment, *Journal of Pediatrics, 77,* 976–985 (1970).

Sameroff, A.J., and Chandler, M.J. Reproductive risk and the continuum of caretaking casualty. In *Review of Child Development Research,* Vol. 4, J.D. Horowitz, M. Hetherington, S. Scarr-Salapatek, and G. Siegel, eds. University of Chicago Press, Chicago (1975).

Siegel, E., Bauman, K.E., Schaefer, E.S., Saunders, M.M., and Ingram, D.D. Home and hospital support during infancy: Impact on maternal attachment, child abuse and neglect, and health care utilization. *Pediatrics, 66,* 183–190 (1980).

Stayton, D.J., Hogan, R., and Ainsworth, M.D.S. Infant obedience and maternal behavior: The origins of socialization reconsidered. *Child Development, 42,* 1057–1069 (1971).

Stern, D. The first relationship: Infant and mother. In *The Developing Child,* J. Bruner, M. Cole, and B. Lloyds, eds. Harvard University Press, Cambridge, Mass. (1977).

White, R. Motivation reconsidered: The concept of competence. *Psychological Review, 66,* 297–333 (1959).

3

Father-Infant Bonding and
the Role of the Father in Child Rearing

Charles E. Hollingsworth

The father-infant bond is just as important as the much publicized mother-infant bond. From the time that conception is recognized, the father begins to develop attitudes toward the pregnancy and fetus that will affect his later inter-actions with the infant. Initially, the expectant father may feel anxiety about the development of the fetus. If the pregnancy was unplanned, ambivalent feel-ings about the pregnancy must be resolved. As the pregnancy progresses, most fathers develop a sense of extreme pride and become very involved with the preparation for delivery. Most men are now very eager to attend parent-infant education classes as well as classes to prepare the couple for labor and delivery. Many couples attend La Maz classes, which tend to bring them closer together and emphasize that this is a mutually satisfying event. The husband becomes a coach and gives emotional support to his wife during the birthing process. Almost all delivery rooms now encourage the husband to be present at the birth of his children. If an emergency develops and the planned vaginal delivery is changed to a cesarean section, only a few hospitals allow the father to go into the operating room. Whenever possible, we encourage hospitals to allow the father into the operating room for his wife's cesarean section, so that he too can see and hold the baby as soon as possible. The father-infant bond is strengthened if the father is present at the delivery. The father is made to feel very important. He acquires precious memories to carry with him throughout the child's life. If the father is not present at delivery, he becomes a captive to his fantasies of what the experience was like for his wife. A father gets the same emotional gratification as the mother of hearing the baby's first cry.

The father should be allowed to room-in with his wife and newborn infant. The father needs to be educated by the nursing staff about all aspects of the infant's care, just as the mother has been traditionally educated. The nursing staff should become more assertive about asking fathers to be present when educational-instructional sessions are held. We strongly encourage the use of the alternate birth room at a well-equipped hospital, with a neonatal intensive care unit nearby in case the infant is in distress. We strongly oppose home deliveries, which are associated with a much higher risk for the infant.

Fathers also benefit from attending classes on how to discipline the child at each developmental stage. A good course in normal child development will alleviate some of the anxiety accompanying the first parenthood. The real task of being an effective, respected, loving parent has barely begun with a successful delivery. Next come years of learning, adjustments, trial and error, and compromises.

The bond between a father and his child is just as crucial for the progress of normal child development as the maternal-infant bond. The father who abdicates his responsibility of parenting his child is depriving the child of emotional security, for which the child must somehow compensate.

Much has been written about the vital importance of the mother-child relationship in the first year of life. The foundation of all future trust and sense of security is laid down as the mother meets the physical and emotional needs of the child. These feelings are the basis for the development of self-esteem, an essential element if a child is to mature into an adult able to love, work, and play without too many problems.

It has always been taken for granted that during this period the father contributes indirectly to the child's well-being by giving the mother emotional support. By being loving, patient, and comforting he helps the mother satisfy the infant's needs. Of course, there have always been fathers who have participated in the baby's physical care—feeding, bathing, changing diapers, and so on. I do not believe that one must be female to be "mothering" to a small infant; a father can exercise the same tender, loving care—and should.

In the case of a newborn child, fathers who refuse to relinquish their primary hold on the mother's attention and who compete actively for her love may seriously impair the emotional development of their child. The father has a responsibility to note and adjust to the changes in his relationship with his wife as children become part of the family.

Fathers make a direct and essential contribution to the child's development. While the helpless infant must be fed, allowed to sleep, and kept warm and comfortable in order to grow emotionally and intellectually, s/he also needs the stimulation of close human contact. By their active participation, fathers, as well as mothers, give the baby that needed stimulation. Fathers enhance the baby's experience with a contact that differs from what the mother provides. When the father holds his infant, it feels different to the child from when the mother holds him. Daddy looks different, sounds different, smells different. He provides the child with variety. A baby needs to hear a deep voice, to sense the way a man handles him or her. It is often Daddy who swings his child into the air or rides him on his shoulders. When Daddy walks into the house, the child's face lights up; something new and exciting is being added to his daily routine. Because the infant has different experiences with his father and mother, he relates differently to each parent. This early variety enriches the child's capacity for warmth, feeling, and responsiveness to other people.

In the first few months of life, children often show a preference for one parent. When Daddy picks them up, they may whimper; and when they are handed to mother, they may relax contentedly. If mother is the preferred parent, many fathers infer that they are not important in their child's life at that stage. Some fathers retreat to fantasies of the time when they will be able to do things with their child—tell him or her a story, teach him or her to swim.

Fathers, like mothers, get real pleasure when the baby smiles at them or imitates sounds they make. The father can help the baby settle down for the night or in other ways give the comfort and security needed. The father becomes even more important to the baby in this regard if the mother suffers from a post-partum depression or psychosis.

The first tooth, the first step, the first word—all the signs of physical and intellectual growth indicating that the child has started on the path of indepen-dent functioning—give parents joy. One of the most important steps in a child's development is his increasing awareness that he is a separate individual, apart from his mother and father. During the second and third years of life, this gradual process erupts into the negativism of the "terrible twos." The "No" which is so characteristic of the two-year-old is his way of demonstrating that he has a will and a mind separate from his mother's or father's. Often, both parents and child have mixed feelings about this independence, desiring yet fearing it. Father's presence and his active contact with the child can encourage the child's independence and present a balance, lessening the chances of a child's remaining tied to his mother.

During the period of "civilizing" the child (toilet training, weaning from breast or bottle, and establishing the myriad other restrictions that eventually transform the demanding, self-centered little king of the universe into a social being, father can participate with mother, upon whom many of these demanding tasks fall. In so doing, he can give his child the opportunity to see that, like mother, Daddy not only satisfies, but also frustrates his needs. Children often have difficulty accepting Daddy's ending a fun activity with them, just as they do when the mother has to end a game with them. These experiences help the child view his parents realistically, ultimately seeing each of them as neither all good nor all bad.

Fatherhood is meant to be a deeply satisfying experience. Few things are more emotionally rewarding than the delight a man gets from satisfactorily guiding his children from birth, through their various stages of development, until they are off on their own.

Every father, whether he is aware of it or not, functions as a child psychologist (Dodson, 1974). He must understand the psychology of his children in order to guide them wisely. If he does not know the vast psychological difference between a three- and a four-year-old, how can he possibly discipline the two ages in an intelligent fashion? Being a good father is determined by the quality rather than the quantity of time spent with children.

Permanent role reversal of the spouses occurs in some families. It may be mutually satisfactory to the parents. Usually, it provides a challenge to children to adopt a model that will allow them to adapt to the society of our next generation. This will be more acceptable as society moves more toward psychosocial gender equality.

REFERENCE

Dodson, F. *How to Father,* J. Harris, ed. Signet, New York (1974).

4

The Pros and Cons of the Alternate Birth Room and the Dangers of Home Deliveries

Katherine F. Carson

Parental attachment to the infant is probably more important to the survival of the species than is medical care. Infants die or develop with difficulty if given only food, warmth, and protection. Babies need intimate involvement with other human beings for their immediate survival and long-term emotional health. The widespread disturbance in parenting and the fragmentation of families in the United States suggest the need for reexamination of those medical practices that affect the involvement of parents with their children. Maternity hospital routines were established before recent research in pediatrics, anthropology, developmental psychology, and physiology created a new appreciation of the remarkable capacities of the neonate for social interaction and of the importance of the neonatal period for a parent-infant involvement. The survival value of these capacities suggests that they are the product of evolutionary selection and must not be lightly discarded. We need to formulate maternity hospital policy to foster positive early parent-infant involvement as well as to prevent some physical complications of childbirth.

There is a growing body of evidence that the advances in decreasing mortality and morbidity by preventing infection and managing physical problems inadvertently altered the initiation of the mother-infant relationship and that some mother-infant pairs may be strained beyond the limits of their adaptability. The routine postpartum separation of healthy mothers and infants appears to approach the limit of minimal contact below which disruptions occur for some mothers. There is now clear evidence that certain maternity hospital practices interfere with breast-feeding and early maternal affection. Controlled studies in four countries demonstrate that hospital routines that separate mother and infant and delay nursing after birth are associated with breast-feeding for a shorter period of time. In the last 10 years in the United States, rooming-in has increased. In a recent survey by Ross Laboratories (Martinez and Nalezienski, 1979) the percentage of infants breast-fed in hospitals went from 24.7 in 1971 to 46.6 in 1978, and those still breast-fed at six months from 5.5 to 20.5 percent. This may be a direct result of rooming-in.

Breast-feeding is not the only response that changes with separation. Specific responses quickly develop between mother and neonate if given the experience of repeated contact. The infant more readily organizes his cycles of sleeping, waking, and crying if exposed to a single caregiver in the first 10 days of life. The day-night rhythm is more quickly established than in infants in a traditional nursery with multiple caregivers and four-hour feeding schedules. The mother who has been with her baby also feels more self-confident and makes fewer calls for advice from medical personnel during the first week at home.

Parental attachment has been shown to depend upon early hospital routines. Attachment is defined as a learned, affectional, and enduring tie to the infant that develops as a result of the interaction with the infant and is shaped by the individual characteristics of the infant, the characteristics and life history of the mother, and the interactions that the mother and infant have with others. The best-studied variable has been that of the influence of the early physical contact between mother and newborn. Early mother-infant separation was linked with subsequent child abuse (Bishop, 1971; Fanaroff, Kennell, and Klaus, 1972). M. Klaus (1972), in his work on bonding, simply let a mother hold her baby skin to skin for 15 minutes within the first hour after delivery, and then compared maternal behaviors 36 hours later regarding measures of attachment: smiling at infant, close contact, encompassing, holding infant, affectionate touch, kissing infant, and looking *en face*. Those who had "bonded" scored much higher than those who had not. A subsequent study comparing a wrapped baby with skin-to-skin contact showed no difference in subsequent maternal behavior as long as the timing was the same (Curry, 1979).

These results should be considered in designing "a birth environment which is physically safe and at the same time considers the psychological well-being of the family unit," as stated in a resolution of the American Nurses Association in June, 1978. But this is not the route by which alternative birth centers came into being. Instead, they resulted from the consumer demand for this type of service.

Over 100 years ago these psychological needs were met by the delivery of most babies at home by an experienced though untrained female midwife. But the maternal and perinatal infant mortality was horrendous. In 1900 in the United States, 500 mothers died for every 100,000 babies born. In 1978, less than 20 die per 100,000. This is because male obstetricians fought tradition and cultural taboos to attend the woman in childbirth and brought scientific medical knowledge and technology to improve her safety and that of her baby. This changed the scene from a familiar bedroom with friends and relatives to a strange-looking hospital room with uniformed, masked nurses and doctors, all others being legally ousted in the name of infection control. Birth became mystified because women no longer participated in any other woman's birth, and perhaps not even in their own if drugged or under general anesthesia. Even though mortality statistics were reduced and birth was safer, women became more afraid because it was the unknown.

To reduce women's panic, childbirth education classes grew up in the United States in the sixties. Birth was once again demystified, but this time the teaching included the husband as a labor coach. The "awake and aware" parturient, as well as her husband, found many things objectionable in the routine treatment of shaving, enemas, intravenous fluids, drugs, and anesthesia, as if she were a production line instead of having a life experience giving birth to their child. The woman specifically objected to the husband being banned from the room while such things were being done, especially if labor was active and she depended on his coaching. More vehemently, women wanted to hold their baby right away, touch it, keep it with them, instead of sending it off to the nursery. They would often present medical reasons to the medical personnel, such as promoting breast-feeding or antibodies in the colostrum, but the truth is that they just wanted to hold the baby. Dr. LeBoyer (1975) interested them in a quiet, darkened environment with a warm water bath that would make the baby open its eyes and respond to eye contact with the parents. They objected to the silver nitrate that closed its eyes to all eye contact.

Instead of responding to this consumerism demand, the hospital delivery suite became technologically even more advanced and began to look like a surgical intensive care unit, with external and even internal fetal monitors, tokodynamometers, continuous epidural anesthesia, and always an intravenous drip, occasionally with pitocin on a pump infusion. The baby was immediately transferred to an expensive warmer, with the heat controlled perfectly for observation, usually out of the sight of the mother. Excellently trained nurses were often more sophisticated in all this equipment than the occasional obstetrician. The higher cesarean section rate complicated the picture even more. The maternal and perinatal mortality went lower and lower, while the cost went higher and higher.

Almost as a contradiction, the same hospitals began to furnish certain labor rooms as alternative birth centers. The appearance is that of a bedroom at home, but emergency equipment for delivery is either hidden there or quickly available nearby. It is a few steps from a regular delivery room or cesarean section room with the team that that procedure requires. The main characteristic is not the cozy appearance, but the change in rules. The woman can have anyone with her she likes (provided they do not have a contagious illness), including her other children. Either midwives or physicians deliver her there, and the baby is not taken from her unless its condition demands it. She may stay there for a few hours while being checked for bleeding and the baby is being checked for temperature and general condition, and then go home, with extra nursing follow-up care, or stay in the usual postpartum suite for several days. Shaving, enemas, intravenous fluids, even monitoring are not required. If observation discloses a problem, she is near a place where it can be solved by running down the hall instead of transferring by ambulance. Some alternative birth centers are free standing and do not have this last advantage, and are therefore a compromise on safety. In some, reduced rates are given, but not in all.

Some disadvantages in this type of delivery are inevitable. Observation cannot be as close if the patient is walking about the room instead of being on a fetal monitor, but this should be acceptable in a low-risk group of mothers. A really high-risk mother is not allowed to use this room. Because of the lack of sterile technique, there is more risk of infection. The friends and relatives also increase the risk of infection. But if no forceps or other invasive techniques are used, infection is reduced anyway. Early discharge has its attendant problems of pediatric follow-up on bilirubin levels and PKU tests, but if the parental attachment has been successful, the parents should follow through on instructions. The backache of the obstetrician leaning over the low bed to repair the perineum is yet to be solved. Although this delivery is designed to meet psychological needs, or at least demands, it may produce problems we do not yet recognize, such as its effect on siblings present. This may be beneficial or harmful, or may depend on variables. Compared with the sibling witnessing a disastrous birth at home, it would seem superior.

Home delivery is the alternative that many parents are choosing to get what they want, partly because they are unaware of what is available in the alternative birth centers. Today, with antibiotics, blood transfusions, and general clenliness, home deliveries could not return to the awesome maternal and fetal mortality of 1900. Today the main causes of maternal mortality are still hemorrhage, infection, and toxemia. Except in sudden disasters, the mother could probably be transported to the hospital in time for lifesaving treatment, but this is not true for the infant. The statistics already show perinatal mortality to be two to five times higher in out-of-hospital deliveries in 11 states, as reported by the American College of Obstetrics and Gynecology. In California, data shows 25 stillbirths per 1000 births for out-of-hospital deliveries, as opposed to 9.9 stillbirths per 1000 births in the hospital. This is even worse, since those who deliver at home are supposed to be only low-risk mothers. Proponents of home delivery say that the statistics for out-of-hospital deliveries also include those who did not plan home delivery but did so inadvertently or on the way to the hospital. This is surely counterbalanced by those who intended to deliver at home, but after three days of neglected labor came to the hospital to deliver the stillborn.

Death is not the only danger. Without fetal monitoring equipment other than a stethoscope, fetal distress cannot be recognized as early. The live baby born in respiratory distress, then further stressed by a chilly trip to the hospital emergency room, may live on with permanent brain damage from anoxia that could have been avoided. Even the best obstetricians can only predict half of the babies that may have distress. Untreated Rh problems, neonatal jaundice from other causes, and unrecognized respiratory problems can take their toll. National statistics that would be reduced by the newer efforts in the hospital deliveries may be increased by the mortality of the home deliveries; the United States will still not be number one in perinatal mortality. Yet, those who succeed in having a healthy baby at home may be rewarded with better parental attachment and a healthier family relationship for the next twenty years (Hirsch, 1979; Wegman, 1979).

Better parental attachment is probably not the motive of those who choose attended or medically unattended home births. Safety is not their main reason, although some will cite the low mortality rates in Holland, where home delivery by a midwife is the norm. Cost is not a factor; the poor still seek hospital care, and midwives as well as doctors charge $1000 or more to deliver at home.

What then are the reasons for home delivery? A child psychiatrist, Richard L. Cohen, M.D., from the University of Pittsburgh School of Medicine, in a recent study of alternative birth centers (personal communication, 1979) concluded that there is a significant and growing population of men and women who do not want childbirth to be a "medical event," and who want to determine how they will have their offspring. They seem willing to incur a modest risk medically in order to do so outside the routinized defensive medicine practice of the modern hospital. In a 1960-1974 study of 300 home birth families, Lubic (1975) reports that only 10 percent of these were counter culture. Ninety percent were straightforward middle class, attended college, owned their own autos and TVs, and often their own homes. We are not dealing with a passive, accepting, unquestioning population, but with knowledgeable young people who are willing to develop their own resources. Many couples choose to bypass the hospital in order to have unlimited contact between mother and child after birth, greater father involvement and personal control of the labor and delivery. Some treasure the experience of home birth for its warm human closeness, others infuse it with spiritual overtones. They say things like: "It just fits into our life style. We try to do things naturally." "Parents are in control and allowed to do things most hospitals forbid." They expect delivery to be a "moment of ecstasy rather than a time of forced labor and pain endured in strange surroundings." They seek a warm, calm, atmosphere, with people around to make the mother feel secure. A typical expression of this attitude is found in a publication of Womancare (1979), a feminist women's health center (San Diego), as follows:

> We found that it was only at home that a woman really had control of her childbirth experience. It was only at home that she could demand and obtain things such as no episiotomy, to hold her baby immediately after birth, and to have those people that she trusted and loved with her at all

times. To be able to help women gain this control became the focus of our childbirth program.

In the publication they then illustrated the contrast between hospital and home delivery, as shown in Fig.

Dr. Richard Cohen has pleaded (personal communication, June 1979):

Child psychiatry and pediatrics have a large and legitimate interest in childbirth care. There is much evidence to suggest that the emotional and mental state of the mother impact both on fetal development and subsequent interaction with the infant, and that these early beginnings are an important factor contributing to the nature of later development.

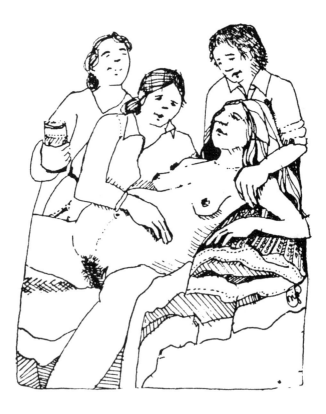

Figure 4.1 Home birth.

In this synthetic modern world young people are grasping at the birth experience as something real that they do not want taken away from them. But home
delivery is likely to give only the realities of damage and death. For their safety,
hospitals must respond to the demands that would contribute to parental attachment, and whenever possible provide parents with a home-style delivery within
the hospital.

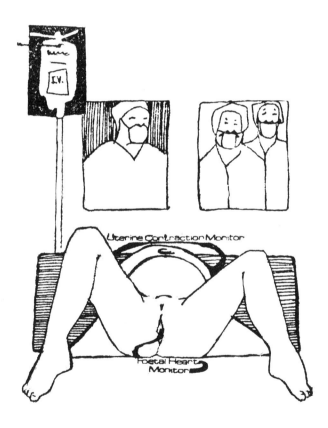

Figure 4.2   Hospital birth.

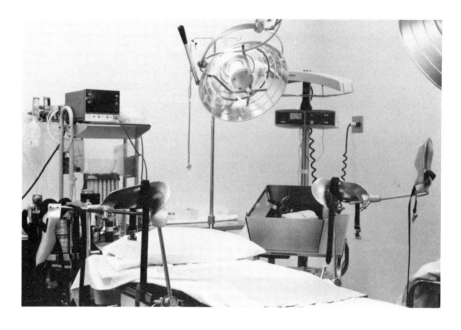

Figure 4.3 Traditional Delivery Room

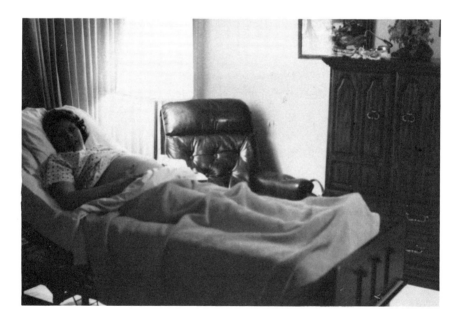

Figure 4.4a Alternate Birth Center in Hospital

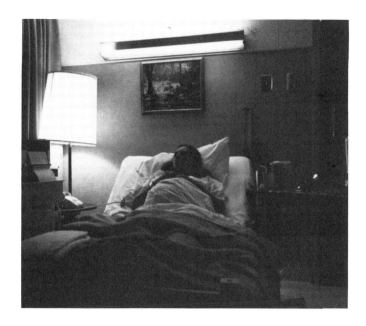

Figure 4.4b Alternate Birth Center Delivery Room

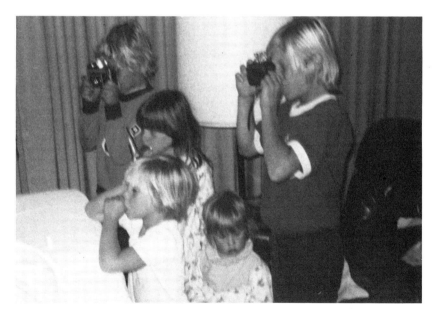

Figure 4.4c The entire family can be included at time of delivery or immediately after delivery.

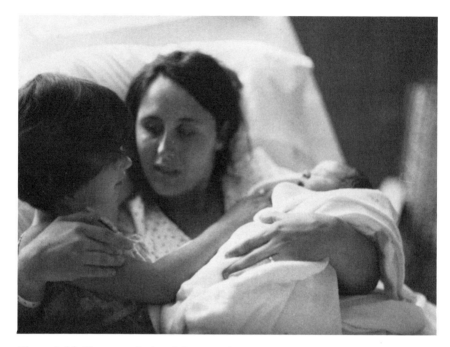

Figure 4.4d If parents desire siblings can be brought in immediately after delivery.

REFERENCES

Bishop, F. Children at risk. *Medical Journal of Australia, 1,* 623–38 (1971).

Cohen, Richard L. Personal Communication (1979).

Curry, A.H. Contact during the first hour with the wrapped or naked newborn: effect on maternal attachment behavior at 36 hours and 3 months, *Birth and the Family Journal, 6,* 227–233 (1979).

Farnoff, A., Kennell, J., and Klaus, M. Follow-up of low birth weight infants— the prediction value of maternal visiting patterns. *Pediatrics, 49,* 288–90 (1972).

Hirsch, H.A. Risks of hospital birth in relation to home birth. *Gynaekologische Rundschau, 19,* Suppl. 2, 18–20 (1979).

Klaus, M. Maternal attachment: Importance of the first post-partum days. *New England Journal of Medicine, 286,* 460–463 (1972).

LeBoyer, F. *Birth Without Violence.* Alfred A. Knopf, New York (1975).

Lubic, R.W. Developing maternity services women will trust. *American Journal of Nursing, 75,* 1685–1688 (1975).

Martinez, G.A., and Nalezienski, J.P. The recent trend in breast feeding (from Ross Laboratories, Columbus, Ohio). *Pediatrics, 64,* 686–692 (1979).

Wegman, M.E. Annual summary of vital statistics for 1978. *Pediatrics, 64,* 835–842 (1979).

Womancare of San Diego. Newsletter. San Diego, Calif. (July 1, 1979).

5

Nursing Considerations in the Alternate Birth Room, in the Normal Neonatal Nursery, and in Rooming-in

Judith Trunecek

Birth is the first-child-parent interaction. It is the culmination of months of development, both for the child and for the expectant parent(s). In the short time attendant to the actual event, we see the personalities, attitudes, concepts, and history of several unique individuals mesh into a unit with but a single purpose—the safe and meaningful birth of another human being.

The mobility of our society and the disruption of the extended family have had an impressive, easily identifiable impact on the childbearing population in this country. There is frequently a noticeable lack of authentic support persons for the pregnant woman. There are, at times, no mother or sister in close proximity, no ever-constant best friend, no well-intentioned neighbor, and sometimes, no father of the child. In contrast, for some parental teams (mother and father) this may be a preplanned, well-rehearsed undertaking in which they function as support for each other.

Ideally, this is a planned for, wanted, eagerly anticipated child who has had the benefit, even *in utero*, of the positive communicative and supportive efforts of a mother and father. Realistically, we may be faced with a juvenile, who is little more than a child herself, trying to cope with an adult situation without benefit of a support person or with one who is as young as she is and knows little of the birthing process and parenting. We may also share the birth experience with the single parent who struggles to show the "world" that she is capable of handling the situation "all by herself," or with the married couple in which only one member wants to include another person in his/her life. Into this potpourri of human beings caught up in the birthing process we place the nurse. Here is the individual who is justifiably proud of the advances in perinatal/neonatal medicine that have in recent history totally reversed the statistics on maternal and neonatal mortality and morbidity. Here is the professional who, in tandem with the physician, provides the knowledge and expertise of practice to the endeavor. The role of the nurse in the alternate birth room and the neonatal nursery must remain one of a concerned, caring, nonjudgmental, supportive individual who is totally attuned to the family unit and its needs and who blends these skills with knowledge and expertise to provide an atmosphere that is supportive to the ultimate awakening of a satisfactory bond between parent(s) and child.

THE ALTERNATE BIRTH ROOM

The parent or parents seeking an alternate birth delivery most commonly fall into two groups. One group consists of those parents who wanted to deliver their child in their own home, with family and friends in attendance. For these, there is a degree of comfort in their own environment. However, after studying all aspects of such a delivery, they decide on delivering in the hospital, where equipment and personnel are available for any emergency that may develop. The second group consists of those parents who always planned delivery in the hospital but wanted conditions that would simulate those of home, with equipment hidden from view, but readily available, and parental control of who will attend the delivery as well as how it will happen. The common denominator for both groups is the welfare of mother and baby.

Attention must be paid to all the details that will be accommodative to the parents' wishes (i.e., a homelike setting; draperies on the windows; paintings on the walls; a big armchair for dad; rugs on the floor; equipment hidden from view in dressers or armoires; a standard single or double bed with a festive coverlet; the lights turned low or the light from a candle illuminating the scene; soft music; the scent of their favorite incense; a glass of wine and a small meal of bread, cheese, and fruit after the advent of the brand new person). Conditions such as these can contribute to the parent(s) feeling of well-being. However, the most important adornment of any alternate birth room is the positive and realistic attitude of the nurse in attendance. The nurse becomes a member of the parent-professional team. Usually, alternate birthing necessitates a one-on-one assignment. The nurse must be allowed time to develop effective, communicative rapport with the parent(s). The nurse needs to be able to spend unspecified amounts of time with the parent(s)—be that 5 minutes or 60. The unrushed acceptance of the parent(s) and the concerns and demands they put forth does more for the emotional acceptance of the situation and task at hand than any other single factor. Nurse and parent must feel good with each other. No question is unreasonable and no explanation is unacceptable. Those nurses who cannot be accepting of this verbal and emotional give and take should not be in the alternate birth room, and their talent should be put to use in a more conventionally acceptable situation. Likewise, parents who cannot give credence to the value of the professional outlook and experience should be hesitant to use the alternate birth room. This is one game in which all the players have to be on the same side, respecting each other and willing to compromise; or else, even in victory there are seeds of discontent. If the nurse keeps the parental and family unit in the foreground, then even if problems develop the parent(s) will still see their needs as being met, and feelings remain positive. If handled in the positive and forthright manner necessary, with recognition of and explanation to the parent(s), the birth experience remains positive. All the important aspects of the birth have been considered and now the unplanned for problem can be dealt with realistically.

Due to the fact that we have a more widely read, informed public via media presentations, self-help books, and parenting and childbirth preparation classes, we also have a group that responds guiltily when things do not proceed just as they did in the book or as the educator said they should. The parent(s) should never plan the child's birth with such adamant expectations that they cannot adapt to the changes that may need to be made in this most natural human experience for the protection and welfare of both mother and child. The changes in plans are less traumatic and guilt producing if there is acceptance of the premise that even in the most low-risk, well-planned, and well-prepared birth there may be a natural element that necessitates giving up one "perfectly" planned moment for a lifetime of acceptable perfection. Parents, in addition to choosing an alternate birth—with labor and delivery in the same bed, with dad and siblings in attendance, with stars and moon in place in the heavens—must also plan alternatives. The parent(s) should come prepared to make the subtle changes that protect the moment and yet allow the medical or natural necessities to be taken care of. If so armed with alternatives, then parents need never feel disappointed in the way things went; for the alternatives were also of their own choosing, but were realistic in their support of the professional management, which is why the alternate birth room was chosen in the first place.

The nurse completes this process of reconciliation with events by being kind, generous, and fair. And when all is over, the parent and the professional can sit back and cooperatively indulge in the joy that is so purely that of a newly born child.

THE NEONATAL NURSERY

Nurseries are meant to be happy, open places enveloped in a protective environment. Certain guidelines are necessary in order to protect the child from infection and disease and to guarantee its general well-being. Thus temperature and draft regulation, curtailment of traffic flow, constant handwashing, and special clothing requirements are standards of care in all nurseries. However, more than anything else, nurseries are meant to be family places. Parents are part of the scheme and should never be considered as visitors. The parent(s) should be encouraged to be active participants in the care of their child.

The majority of all newborn infants will be able to go to their mother's room shortly after birth. They can become rapidly initiated into the world of the family. The concept of family-centered care allows the parent(s) to participate in all aspects of the child's care in a controlled setting that has numerous resource persons to answer questions or intervene directly. This is the time when the family gets to know each other. Bonding of parent and child is begun, with emphasis on quality as well as quantity.

The nursery nurse must be more than a caretaker. Teaching, both formal and informal, is one of the primary functions involved in the care of the newborn infant. Usually, the parent is a receptive, concerned, and somewhat frightened student. The nurse must be willing to share her knowledge and experience in a way that is both understandable and relevant to the parent(s). After researching the needs of a particular family, the needed information can be presented faithfully and supportively. The nurse must be willing to invest time and patience to achieve a satisfactory result. An accepting, nonthreatening attitude is a necessity.

Parental acceptance and comfort is more threatened in those instances in which the child is ill after birth, or is premature, or small for gestational age. The normal time allowed in both delivery suite and nursery for child-parent bonding may be severely curtailed or even nonexistent initially. Even the most advised parent(s) do not ever plan for anything other than a perfect child. This places the nurse in a unique position. More than any other health professional, the nurse can help facilitate bonding and general parenting by encouraging the parent(s) to participate as fully as possible in the care of the child, even if this may mean only holding the child's hand for a few minutes each time the parent comes to visit. Touching is a very positive form of communication for these parents, and equipment need not be a deterrent to involvement. However, the nurse must always be respectful of the parents as individuals with needs and feelings and proceed at a pace that is acceptable to both.

Often, being an interested observer is reassuring to the parent. If the baby spits up, turns blue, or fusses for the nurse (a professional), it then becomes acceptable for these things to happen to the parent also. Knowing the community resources available to the parent(s) is also an invaluable tool. The cooperation between the nursery nurse and the unit social worker can spell the difference between the ultimate success or failure for the parent. Adjustments to assimilate the new baby into the already existing lifestyle can be made with relative ease when the parent knows the options.

Positive interaction between nurse and parent can remarkably improve the outcome for any infant. The resultant parental assurance can serve as a positive force in the future of both parent and child.

In summary, the nurse in the perinatal/neonatal setting can be a resource, teacher, helper, caretaker, and companion for the modern parent. In respecting parental ideas, needs, and aspirations, the nurse can serve as a catalyst in the encounter that sets in motion a new human being on that greatest of adventures —life.

ROOMING-IN

Rooming-in is that traditional concept whereby the mother and her newborn baby are guaranteed time to be together. The facilities provided to achieve this vary widely with each hospital, but an aware, participative nursing staff does not. This is a shared time period for nurse, parent, and baby, which, if used properly, greatly enhances the adjustment of baby to the family and to family life. It is a time for questions, honest answers, and comfort. How the parent perceives the idiosyncrasies of caring for the baby influences the general acceptance of both the normal and problematic aspects of infant care. The nurse can readily key in on problem areas and can then arrange for the proper support. This support may range from a complete social service workup to a simple matter of just being available to the parent to answer questions or to intervene directly.

During this "getting-to-know-you" period the mother and father learn about baby care. With a resource person, helper, or supervisor in attendance or readily available, the parent learns to feed, bathe, pamper, and accept the child for what it is—a unique individual.

In present-day maternity care, this concept has been elaborated to assume an aspect that is particularly geared toward fostering the family. No longer is father excluded from active care of the new child. He is encouraged to come to the hospital as a parent, not as a visitor. He actively participates in the life of the mother and baby during hospitalization and learns to feed, change diapers, communicate with, and quiet the new infant. Mother and father learn to assume and cooperate on aspects of caretaking, but also have time to learn about each other in this new role and how they can best adjust to this new being.

Consideration must be given to the mother and child to provide an experience that is meaningful and yet realistic. Expectations of both parent and child should not be so high as to prime them for failure. Recognition of parental needs is not contrary to the achievement of quality bonding. Many parents exhibit a sense of failure if faced with a baby who may be problematic. This is one area in which there are few absolutes, and the professional does his client a service if alternative positive behaviors are expressed and allowed. If the mother is tired, she must be helped to see that it is acceptable if she needs to rest and therefore cannot feed the baby this time. The father can help transcend the difficult times if he also is made to feel comfortable with the child.

Rooming-in, or family-centered care, can help the parent and child through the initial period of adjustment and will help build parental assurance and child comfort. In essence, it serves as in-service training for the home-bound family.

6

High-Risk Infant Follow-up

Kristin Gist

Follow-up studies of the high-risk neonate have typically focused upon the intellectual status of the child, without comment upon the use of the assessment as a kind of intervention in itself (Lubchenco, 1972; Drillien, 1972; Pape et al., 1978). Studies have typically been available only when funded by large grants and therefore tend to be found only in large university hospital systems.

This chapter focuses on the feasibility of a relatively inexpensive follow-up program that serves not only to evaluate the developmental outcome of the high-risk neonate, but also to optimize the development of the high-risk infant and simultaneously facilitate the affectional attachment between parents and infant.

The high-risk infant is defined here as one who graduates from the neonatal intensive care unit and meets one or more of the following criteria: birth weight of less than or equal to 1500 grams, neonatal asphyxia (infant requires active resuscitation in the delivery room and/or has a one-minute Apgar of less than 5 or a five-minute Apgar of less than 7), respiratory distress syndrome, small for gestational age, bilirubin greater than 20 milligrams percent. The criteria might be expanded to include teenage mothers, prenatal drug abuse, genetic defects, etc., depending on the needs of the institution.

PURPOSE OF THE EVALUATION

There are a number of clinical purposes in evaluating the development of the high-risk infant. The first is to provide reassurance to the parents that their infant is developing normally. Second, the evaluation can identify developmental delay at an early age and provide avenues for remediation. Third, the evaluation can serve as a teaching tool for normal developmental expectations. And fourth, the evaluation can serve to provide parents with a better understanding of their infant's temperament and learning style.

WHEN TO EVALUATE DEVELOPMENT

Testing has been done in the Neonatal Follow-up Developmental Evaluation Clinic at Children's Hospital and Health Center, San Diego, California, at the following ages: 6 months, 12 months, 24 months, 3½ years, 5 years, and 7 years. Ages for evaluation were determined with consideration for the infant's needs, the parents' needs, and the examiner's capabilities regarding time and number of children. Optimally, infants would first be examined at term by use of the Brazelton Neonatal Behavioral Assessment Scale, with parents present, and then seen after a predetermined period at home. Routine follow-up examinations done at three months were discontinued, as too many infants continued to show disorganization and developmental delays, which were resolved by six months. The evaluation itself seemed to contribute to parents' anxiety regarding the infant's capabilities; therefore, the examiner's "interference" was determined as detrimental to an already tenuous parent-infant relationship, regardless of the care taken by the examiner to provide parental support.

A routine 18-month evaluation was eventually also omitted from the program because of heightened separation anxiety and control issues, which interfered with a valid examination. Language is the area most often of concern at this age, yet language could not be directly assessed, as the child was quiet when around a stranger. Testing was equally difficult at home or in the hospital setting. Eighteen-month evaluations are attempted if delay is suspected at 12 months, so that a determination can be made about the need for referral.

The age of three years was determined as a difficult age for evaluation, since boys in particular were observed to become clingy and difficult to separate, yet were not comfortable with difficult items when parents were present. A further difficulty with this age is using the McCarthy Scales of Children's Abilities is that the instrument seems not to back up to the Bayley Scales of Infant Development, and therefore the child with mild delays may not achieve a basal in some areas. This problem is not observed with the Stanford-Binet, as there is an overlap with the Bayley ages.

WHO EVALUATES DEVELOPMENT

Who evaluates the child is determined by the nature of the follow-up clinic, but typically too many disciplines alienate parents as well as community physicians who are providing primary care. The psychologist can provide an excellent overall assessment, as he or she is trained in the integration of all aspects of psychological functioning. The nurse practitioner or public health nurse could administer a screening test, such as the Denver Developmental Screening Test, and refer for more in-depth evaluation as needed.

An appreciation for the examiner's level of competence should be known before one utilizes psychological test reports in making a diagnostic decision. Tests that are administered by students or interns often lack clinical interpretation of the child's behavior responsiveness during the test. The child's relative mood can increase or decrease test scores dramatically. Therefore, in children who are negative, fatigued, shy, or who display a general lack of attention, abilities would not be brought to their best performance by an inexperienced examiner.

Although traditional training in administering standardized psychological tests is a must, a solid foundation in normal child development is of equal importance. Comfort with typical behaviors at each age below four years is essential in drawing a child into his optimal performance. For example, direct questioning of a two-year-old for vocabulary often elicits an emphatic "No," whereas having the toddler "read" the pictures to a baby (a doll) might elicit gleeful cooperation. Likewise, direct inquisition for identification of body parts on a doll often elicits refusal in a 1½-year-old, who is delighted to take a tissue and "wipe the jelly off baby's food." Such play techniques provide parents with new ideas for dealing with their toddler's oppositional behavior as well as some valuable information regarding the child's style of interacting at that point in his or her development.

The disciplines employed for further evaluation of suspected specific disabilities include speech pathology, audiology, occupational therapy, physical therapy, infant educators, and medical specialists.

WHAT INSTRUMENTS ARE USED

There are a number of instruments appropriate for evaluating the infant and young child. The Bayley Scales of Infant Development has three parts: a mental scale, a motor scale, and an infant behavior record. The mental scale is designed to assess perceptual abilities, memory, object permanence, problem solving, language, and the beginning of abstract and symbolic thinking. The motor scale provides assessment of motor development and coordination. The behavior record assists the examiner in assessing the child's social, behavioral, and emotional functioning. The Bayley Scales provides a comprehensive assessment of the child's development, offering many items in the area of cognitive functioning. The materials are varied and colorful and are enjoyed by children and parents. However, because of the many imitative motor tasks, the Bayley is difficult to use with motorically impaired children, particularly prior to the development of language.

The Bayley is the most widely used infant test, particularly in follow-up of high-risk neonates. It is preferred because it has the newest and most representative norms and is constructed so that the clinician can compare the child's functioning in three broad areas (mental, motor, and behavior) to the same sample population. The Bayley has been shown to be a reliable and valid instrument for use with infants, and its concurrent validity is demonstrated by high positive correlations with other infant tests, such as the Gesell and the Cattell.

The Gesell is widely and more appropriately used by pediatricians and is also considered comprehensive, although test scores are particularly affected by children with cerebral palsy, as motor functioning is included in the overall developmental quotient. It provides comprehensive information for use in counseling parents. An advantage of using either the Gesell or the Bayley is that these scales are most widely used in follow-up studies and therefore provide an adequate basis for comparison of data. Other instruments used to evaluate infant development include the Denver Developmental Screening Test, the Merrill-Palmer Scale of Mental Abilities, and the Cattell Infant Intelligence Scale. The Uzgiris and Hunt Ordinal Scales of Psychological Development provide further opportunity for evaluating cognitive processes, and the object permanence scale is easily integrated into the Bayley without a great deal of additional time being involved.

Selection of an instrument used in longitudinal follow-up of the older child depends upon the type of data desired by a particular study. The Stanford-Binet Intelligence Scale, Form L-M, is one of the most widely used measures of intelligence in young children because of the large age range that it covers and because of its extremely good reliability and validity. Its predictive validity (correlation with later academic achievement) is the highest of any preschool measure of general intelligence. This instrument requires a level of verbal response at approximately the two-year level and is not as useful for children with significantly impaired sensorimotor or language skills. However, excellent information can be obtained from use of the Stanford-Binet in conjunction with a nonverbal scale. The Stanford-Binet has the advantage of overlapping in age with the Bayley and provides one measure that can be used consistently to adulthood. The disadvantage of this instrument is in its highly verbal nature and lack of performance items measuring conceptual thinking abilities.

The McCarthy Scales of Children's Abilities covers an age range of 2½ to 8½ years. It is becoming more widely used in follow-up programs. It is divided into six subscales that include 18 subtests, and the general cognitive index, which is derived by combining the verbal, perceptual performance and quantitative scales, is roughly equivalent to the Stanford-Binet I.Q. The McCarthy is most useful with young children who are not retarded but have mild learning deficits. Because it has many different tasks and colorful, interesting materials, it can be good for children who are inattentive and hard to motivate. However, it is quite long and often needs to be administered in two or more sessions. Validity data for this test are incomplete. The motor scale is a helpful addition to this instrument, particularly with the high-risk population.

The Leiter International Performance Scale is a measure of nonverbal intelligence commonly used for hard-of-hearing and language-handicapped children. The tasks require perceptual matching, analogies, memory, and other varied items, many similar to verbal tests. It can be used appropriately in conjunction with the Stanford-Binet or the McCarthy Scales to further define the extent of delayed development with regard to suspected language delay. The *Arthur Adaptation* is the recommended manual for administration; it covers ages 2 through 12 years.

The Weschler tests are not appropriate before age four, and their use necessitates frequent instrument changes.

CONSIDERATIONS TO BE MADE IN TESTING INFANTS

There are special considerations to be taken in evaluating the development of infants and young children, regardless of the instrument used. First is the issue of separation. The young infant, approximately 0–5 months old, can be handled fairly comfortably by strangers and still deliver his best performance. Mother and father, on the other hand, gain no benefit themselves if they are omitted from the testing procedure. Therefore, it is important to test the infant as a part of the family unit.

The 6–12-month-old shows a marked increase in stranger awareness and cannot usually tolerate being handled immediately by the examiner. He interacts nicely, however, if held securely in mother's lap.

The 12–18-month-old is perhaps the most difficult to evaluate because of the fears of separation from the parent. This child can typically be tested in a highchair, with minimal direct interaction, following a period of exploration around the examiner. Because play at this age is object oriented, rapport can be established through toys, and later the level of interaction can be optimal.

The two-year-old generally enjoys the interaction of the testing situation if a parent is present. Complete separation at this age is not smooth, and rapport can be more quickly established with mother's or father's assistance.

The three-year-old seems to become clingy again after a period of independence, particularly the child who did not resolve issues of dependency and control in the second year. This dependent behavior, including difficulty in interacting with the examiner, persists whether or not parents leave the room. The three-year-old who is able to separate (and whose mother is able to separate as well) shows a much higher level of cooperation and motivation than the child whose parent must remain. By 3½ years, most children separate without difficulty and perform better without parents present (i.e., are able to persist on difficult items).

A second consideration in testing young children is to begin with the mother-father-child unit rather than with looking at the child by himself. Observations can be made while the parents utilize toys to make the child feel at ease. Judgment must be withheld, however, for the parent who feels so uncomfortable herself that she cannot be spontaneous in her interactions with her infant.

Positive comments are essential in establishing rapport and setting the parents at ease. Such comments as "What a cute baby!" or "Those overalls are perfect on such a cold day" relieve a formal atmosphere and assist in putting a parent at ease in conversation which is comfortable and familiar. Parents can then be led into conversation about the baby's personality, temperament, sleeping and eating habits, and specific concerns regarding developmental progress.

The physical setting for testing infants and children is crucial in obtaining an optimal response. Testing, whether in home or office, brings the presence of a stranger. Some infants seem more comfortable at home, but this study has found that toddlers who are evaluated in familiar settings have an increased tendency to refuse cooperation and have difficulty in concentrating on the test items if they are able to leave easily. In either event, the testing room should be relatively free from distraction and have only two or three toys in view. It should contain a comfortable table-and-chair arrangement (so that the baby who needs to may sit in mother's lap) and adequate floor space to allow spontaneous movement. A floor pad or crib is necessary for very young infants (0–4 months), and a highchair is helpful for children nine months to three years of age to provide some control over their tendency to leave after each item. Such behavior contributes to fatigue early in the examination, particularly for the distractible infant. A small table-and-chair set is ideal for the older child. Testing in an office is easier when the Bayley Scales of Infant Development are utilized, as they require a standardized set of stairs and balance beam for complete evaluation of psychomotor development.

Timing is an important consideration in children of all ages, but is especially crucial for children under two years. Some judgment must be made in the initial observations regarding the level of direct interaction the child can tolerate. This, plus his level of interest in the first test materials, provide cues about his readiness to begin. Testing sometimes must be interrupted for a rest (some children become easily overstimulated by different materials or by rapid transition), for diaper change, or feeding. At times, particularly with the 2–3-year-old, testing must be aborted altogether because of lack of cooperation. After a concerted effort to end the interaction on a positive note, the appointment should be scheduled for several weeks or months away. Such circumstances as the arrival of a new baby, death in the family, or special holidays interrupt a child's routine and render him unable to adapt to the demands of the evaluation.

Most test materials for children under the age of four (Bayley, Gesell, Merrill-Palmer, Stanford-Binet) are interesting and colorful. As such, they can be presented in a way that gives the child the comfort of playing informal games while maintaining complete accuracy of administration. Picture vocabulary need not be demanded, but can be elicited by mother after brief instructions to her, or "baby doll" can be involved to "listen" while the child "reads" the pictures. Allowing the child to test the psychologist following certain items, such as visual memory, contributes to a gamelike situation that facilitates cooperation.

CLINICAL USES OF THE EVALUATION

The psychological evaluation provides many opportunities beyond the accumulation of test scores and determination of the level of psychological functioning. The session can be used for interpreting a child's temperament to the parent and can offer the parent a new perspective in his interaction with his baby, as illustrated by the following case.

Phillip was born at 29 weeks' gestation and weighed 1100 grams (2 pounds, 7 ounces). He was hospitalized for 46 days with asphyxia, respiratory distress syndrome, and apnea. Phillip was rehospitalized at three months of age following a severe apneic episode. He was from an intact family of four-year-old twin girls and older siblings 15, 17, and 19 years of age. He was reported to be awake and fussy throughout most of the day and night, and by the time of his evaluation at nine months of age (six months adjusted for prematurity), he did not yet nap, nor did he seem to have a routine. He was noted to be a highly distractible infant, mouthing toys excessively, with eyes darting around the room as he reached persistently, not looking at any toy that he obtained. His test scores were average on the Bayley, with a mental development index of 94 and a psychomotor development index of 104. Psychomotor development, however, was highly variable, with early standing, usually on toes, and early mobility, but delayed sitting. Phillip seemed frantic throughout the evaluation and the tendency was to hurry before he crashed. However, his needs were for the examiner to move very slowly, providing few materials at a time, and to offer time without stimulation between items. The table was kept clear of materials so as not to contribute to his visual disorganization. When mother needed to feed Phil, lights were turned off to lower the level of stimulation.

Although the mother was reassured that Phillip was demonstrating age-appropriate developmental milestones, it was suggested that she attempt to provide a low level of stimulation in Phil's everyday environment. He required gentle rhythmic movement in a quiet room rather than talking and bouncing, as the latter caused Phillip to become upset. A total family effort ensued whereby measures were taken to provide a relatively low-key environment for Phil, a difficult feat with six children. The improvement in selective attention and organization was obvious by 12 months, although Phil at two years continues to require much help in achieving a relaxed and organized state. His mother has acquired a new understanding of Phillip's needs and individual differences and has an enhanced self-image as a successful parent. The evaluation provided a medium for teaching about "infant characteristics" such as effectivity, persistence, level of attention, sensitivity, activity, quieting and consolability, and initiation (Huntington, 1979).

TEACHING CHILD DEVELOPMENT

Teaching normal developmental expectations is a useful aspect of the evaluation setting. The potentially abusive parent who overinterprets the infant's behavior can benefit greatly by learning the release of an object at five months is involuntary. Five-month-old Katie's hand was slapped for dropping her mother's keys in the hallway prior to Katie's appointment. Mother needed the information that Katie's hand opened involuntarily as she shifted her attention to toys inside the room. The 9-12-month-old who throws everything on the floor is experimenting with both cause and effect and the release of objects and is learning to appreciate object permanence. However, this behavior is often misconstrued as deliberate and oppositional.

The developing independence observed in the 15-24-month-old can be handled casually and sensitively by the examiner, who provides a model for parents who are terrified of the tantrums and have fear of losing control. The parent can be educated to reinforce patterns of healthy behaviors and thus increase the probability of their occurrence.

PROVIDING FEEDBACK

Perhaps the most sensitive issue in providing developmental evaluations of infants at risk involves interpreting results to the parents. Although certain follow-up programs do not provide feedback as part of their procedure, the danger in not sharing information with the parent is that the parent will leave with the feeling that baby is less than normal, is some kind of specimen to be studied. In the high-risk infant, this is a feeling that occurred initially during the child's neonatal course and, undoubtedly, soon after the child's discharge from the hospital. If this feeling is reinforced at the time of follow-up, this can delay the attachment process. The examiner is faced with the dilemma of interpreting worrisome signs, while facilitating the parent/infant relationship. Scrutinizing the high-risk infant's development calls attention to deviations from normal development which might otherwise go unnoticed and even resolve themselves. The dilemma, then, is in recognizing these signs and conveying information to parents without interrupting an already tenuous attachment process. When an infant from the neonatal intensive care unit goes home to his parents, the parents are often withholding some degree of love and affection, which were designated for the "normal" baby who was not born. This affection is withheld until the high-risk infant begins to show the parents that he is developing. His smile, his focus, his hand play are all signs to parents that the baby is developing normally, and these signs assist in breaking down the wall parents have built to protect themselves from becoming attached.

The follow-up evaluation can strengthen the good feelings that the parent has toward the infant. The psychologist can provide reassurance and support that the baby is moving in a normal direction of growth and development, thus freeing parents from some element of worry and concern, which inhibits their spontaneous joy in play. Parents benefit from having the baby's temperament and style of learning interpreted to them. For example, a baby who is often fussy, who is constantly being jostled and stimulated to curtail crying, might show increased irritability with high levels of stimulation and transitions from one test item to another. If parents can understand what contributes to the irritability, the changes in their own style of handling might yield a calmer, easier infant.

On the other hand, the infant who is quiet, rather passive, and given to long periods of visual inspection prior to smiling or handling objects might be described as dull or delayed by parents who are accustomed to an active, outgoing child. Helping parents appreciate the needs of this child to warm up slowly, while at the same time reassuring them that his or her development is normal, provides invaluable assistance to the mother-father-child unit. Many individual differences (i.e. active and outgoing versus quiet and slow to warm up) are comfortable in one family and disconcerting in another. Interpretations of individual temperament and personality can facilitate acceptance of the child.

SIGNS AND SYMPTOMS OF DELAYED DEVELOPMENT

The following are examples of signs and symptoms that have been observed by this author to sometimes lead to specific developmental disorders. Their appearance early on is not necessarily indicative of the disorder, but is merely suggestive, and is cause for close and careful observation without undue alarm. One symptom is rarely worrisome, but several abnormal responses, which are obligatory, often are significant.

I. Signs that might indicate cerebral palsy
   A. At six months
      1. Early laterality, with nonpreferred hand held in fisted position and/or arm in flexed position
      2. Fine hand tremors
      3. Poor trunk support, rounded back in supported sit
      4. Delay in head control and/or hyperextension of the head and neck
      5. Significant discrepancy between MDI and PDI on the Bayley Scales, with PDI accelerated at six months related to early standing (rigidity in lower extremities); drop in PDI occurs rather quickly after six months as sitting skills are not acquired.
II. Signs suggestive of language disorder
   A. At six months
      1. Delayed localization to sound coupled with normal brainstem evoked response
      2. High distractibility
      3. Increased startle to noise
   B. At 12 months
      1. Increase in activity level with little evidence of receptive language
      2. Delay in auditory attention
   C. At three years
      1. Improved test scores, motivation, and attention span for nonverbal items
      2. Significant discrepancy between nonverbal reasoning tasks and language items
III. Signs suggestive of hyperactivity
   A. At six months
      1. Excessive mouthing
      2. High distractibility
      3. Poor visual organization
      4. Frantic behavior that increases with transitions between test items
      5. Poor sleep patterns
      6. High psychomotor score related to early mobility
      7. Delayed sitting without evidence of cerebral palsy

These lists are quite brief and may be more or less complete after further study. Concerns about such diagnoses as language disorder and hyperactivity could be useful only if they encourage parents to provide some changes in the infant's environment to improve his organizational abilities. For example, in a highly active, distractible, fussy infant, parents might be encouraged to feed this child in a darkened room with low level of stimulation (i.e., away from other family members and without talking and jostling). The six-month-old who appears unusually active often demands higher levels of stimulation, but tolerates only the lower levels. For example, this child might be rocked, but not looked at and talked to simultaneously. Or he might be stroked and looked at, but not talked to.

Depending upon the severity, number of related signs, and parents' readiness, referral or recommendation for referral may or may not be made. Many observed signs of abnormal development resolve spontaneously, as illustrated in the following example.

> Thomas, at six months, demonstrated a predominant right-hand preference, left arm sometimes flexed, left leg and toe hyperextended, toes curled under. Reexamination at eight months demonstrated resolution of the early laterality and only slightly delayed eye-hand coordination; no lower extremity problems were observed. Resolution of these problems occurred presumably because they were minimal and because the mother was given timely information that laterality normally is not well established by six months and that increased input to the left hand would undoubtedly result in more frequent use of it. She had been encouraged to minimize the use of the Jolly Jump-Up, walker, and other activities that reinforced hyperextension of the lower extremities, to allow Thomas to gain mobility and pull to standing on his own. The parents' input may have resolved early signs of mild spasticity.

While similar information is easily assimilated by some, this may be too much for one who is defending. Even such information as the need for a hearing test following delayed localization may be too threatening. The parents' attitude must be considered at least as important as the earliest possible remediation; therefore, no discrepancy in development can be viewed as an emergency unless the parent views it as such.

CONSIDERATION IN PROVIDING PARENTS WITH FEEDBACK REGARDING REAL OR POTENTIAL DELAYS

In evaluating the development of all premature infants, an adjustment in age must be made. This age correction is obtained by subtracting the number of weeks of prematurity from the child's chronological age. While this is felt, at times, to yield an overinflated development index, it is more accurate than disregarding prematurity altogether, particularly for the child who is born very early (i.e. at ≤32 weeks' gestation. At an arbitrary point, age correction must be foregone so that the child can be clinically evaluated with his peers prior to school entrance. This examiner has chosen the age of 2½ to forego the age correction, although an initial drop in test scores is expected.

The only significant issue in prolonged age adjustment regards time of school entrance. If a child's expected delivery date is after the cutoff date for kindergarten entry, there is every reason to delay a child's school entry until the following year. The immaturity of the very young kindergartner, coupled with possibilities of minimal brain dysfunction or delays in attention and organization, contribute to school failure.

Kind of Information Conveyed

Early definitive, predictive information is not only inappropriate, it is impossible to obtain, although the parents' desire to know the long-term outcome at this point must be appreciated and recognized.

Importance of Assessing Parents' Readiness

It is important to assess the parents' readiness for information regarding deviations from normal development. Parents assist in our conveying information by giving us information about how they see their baby developing. Observations from the evaluation must be incorporated into the parents' own observations, and if the parents do not see the child's behavior or development as a problem, then it cannot be a problem for the examiner at that point. The responsibility of the examiner lies in preparing the parents to be more ready at the next evaluation.

An infant whose development is considered problematic in one family can be regarded as normal in another.

> Jimmy was a fussy, disorganized, active baby. His mother was worried because his twin seemed to be developing more rapidly and was calmer and more organized in his play. Linda, too, was a rather distractible, disorganized infant with a high activity level; but her young parents had no other children comparison and were proud of her level of activity and visual alertness.

Assessing Readiness for Referral

Determining a parent's readiness for an agency or program referral is difficult. This readiness is often, but not always, best determined by the pediatrician, if he or she has a close relationship with the family. Parents differ in their readiness for intervention in timing and in kind, and this difference must be recognized.

The parent who is worried about an unusual sign in development will feel better about the baby if he has a specific intervention program and a teacher to help him with the problem, as illustrated in the following example.

Cathy is a triplet who was born two months prematurely and suffered an intracranial hemorrhage resulting in hydrocephalus. She had a normal sister, and a brother who was ill with heart disease and eventually died. Before the death of the brother, when Cathy was six months old (adjusted age), the mother came to the evaluation asking to be referred to a physical therapy program so that she would know the kinds of exercises to do to decrease her daughter's obvious spasticity (although she did not know the terminology). After consultation with the pediatrician, she was referred for neurological consultation, and Cathy has received occupational and physical therapy since six months.

A parent who is not ready for intervention, but feels responsible for the child's degree of delay, needs time and suggestions for working with the baby on her own.

Susie was born at 31 weeks' gestation. A fraternal twin, she had a mild neonatal course when compared with her brother, who had severe RDS, necrotizing enterocolitis, and a patent ductus arteriosus. Susie's primary neonatal problem was poor feeding and apnea of prematurity. Susie's development at six months' adjusted age appeared to be that of developing spastic diplegia. Although Susie's development was not seriously delayed for her age at that point, the prognosis was very poor, as there was already hyperextension of the feet, head, and neck, and fisting of one hand. Gentle interpretation of the significance of these signs brought guilt reactions and defending from the mother, who expressed responsibility for her child's delay. She related that these children were born late in life and that she had not spent as much time with the twins as she had with her earlier children. She vowed to go home, work with the babies, and bring them back in three months, showing that they were normal. This decision by the mother was accepted. Six weeks later the mother called for a re-evaluation, as she was concerned that Susie's problems were becoming more severe and she was ready for help. Allowing the mother time initially, saved time for the infant in the long run.

There may be a time when the mother is ready for intervention, but it may not be in the best interests of the baby at that particular stage of his development.

Michael, who was in foster care, was receiving occupational and physical therapy weekly for his severe psychomotor delay resulting from a spinal defect. Although there was indication for further kinds of therapeutic intervention, he was grappling with issues of independence and control and arguing frequently with his foster mother, who was determined that he perform better and better. At this point, further intervention, such as speech therapy (which would impose more control on this child in an area where he had difficulty performing), would further hamper his motivation and persistence. The period of 18 to 24 months for this child was considered extremely critical, and timing for further intervention would have been poor. In this situation, it was helpful for the mother to understand what Michael's needs were and to establish priorities regarding his personality and development.

The dilemma facing the examiner, then, is one for which there are no clear answers. There is no best age at which an infant's development should be evaluated. Nor is there a set time for making observations of abnormal development or referrals. It seems most important to incorporate information into the parents' own knowledge and observations of the child and to recognize that timing of information and intervention is as essential for the parents' own feelings toward their child as it is for the child achieving optimal development.

HOW FOLLOW-UP INTERFACES WITH THE REST OF THE INSTITUTION AND OUTSIDE AGENCIES

Specialists from within the institution can provide more specific diagnostic information when the parent is ready. The pediatric neurologist, orthopedist, speech pathologist, audiologist, occupational and physical therapists—all provide invaluable information in defining the extent of a child's delayed development. Complete diagnostic information need not be obtained before recommendation of an intervention program, and often a parent must feel some success in remediating delays before achieving readiness to further define the problem. The private pediatrician is often best able to assist in determining a family's coping style and can provide consultation prior to selection of an appropriate agency.

Regional centers, schools, and state and private agencies provide intervention for infants with developmental delay. Care must be taken in selecting a program, with consideration of cost, parents' needs, and specific kinds of delays in development.

INCIDENCE OF HANDICAPPING CONDITIONS IN THE
ICU POPULATION

Many studies provide information regarding the developmental outcome of the intensive care unit (ICU) survivor (Drillien, 1964; McDonald, 1964; Parmelee and Schulte, 1970). This author has followed approximately 900 intensive care unit survivors born since December, 1973. Children presently range in age from neonates to seven years. Certain tendencies in developmental outcome have been observed.

When infants who suffered from respiratory distress syndrome during the neonatal period are evaluated as a group (N = 245), the distribution follows an approximately normal curve and the mean I.Q. is 100. The incidence of handicap increases rapidly when those infants who weigh less than 1500 grams (3 pounds, 4 ounces) are separated from the total. Approximately 28 percent of these infants, who suffered neonatal asphyxia as well as severe respiratory distress syndrome (requiring mechanical ventilation or CPAP), are considered significantly handicapped. Handicapping conditions include cerebral palsy; retrolental fibroplasia, resulting in significant visual loss; and hearing loss. The group of children with severe respiratory distress syndrome and without neonatal asphyxia yield a 25 percent incidence of significant handicapping conditions. Developmental aphasia was also observed, and, as a rule, physical and mental disabilities were less severe. Cerebral palsy was observed most often in the asphyxiated infant.

A diagnosis of recurrent apnea (N = 80) was given to infants who demonstrated apnea and bradycardia that was felt to be more severe and recurrent than that observed in other infants born at the same gestational age. Thirty percent of this group were found to be physically or mentally handicapped, an incidence that is higher than in any other single diagnostic group. Although statistical tests have not yet been performed, handicaps are observed most often in the infant with apnea born at 25–28 weeks of gestation and next in the infant born at 30–32 weeks of gestation.

The number of very small infants, weighing 1000 grams or less (2 pounds, 3 ounces), who survive is rapidly increasing, and with it the number of infants with chronic lung disease. The resulting prolonged hospitalization carries the risk of sensory deprivation, sensory overload, and seriously delayed mother-father-infant bonds, as well as lack of normal handling and motor input. While these infants are at greatest risk for developmental delay and attachment disorders, they also require more time before delays can be determined as significant. For example, cortical blindness was inappropriately diagnosed in an infant who was very slow to begin processing visual information secondary to prolonged hospitalization and immaturity. By 11 months (adjusted age), this child's visual functioning was normal. Similar findings regarding poorly integrated visual responses were reported in 1966 by S. Saint-Anne Dargassies.

Thirty-nine children weighing 1000 grams or less at birth have been studied. The average I.Q. for this group is 83, and the psycomotor development index at the latest evaluation in infancy yielded an average score of 90, compared with a mean of 100. The frequency distribution was observed to be bimodal, with 22 percent of the children having mental scores below 70. The incidence of significant handicapping conditions is approximately 50 percent, and specific disabilities include hearing loss, cerebral palsy, blindness, and mental retardation.

The prognosis for children suffering an intracranial hemorrhage, resulting in hydrocephalus, during the neonatal period is improving. Ten such infants are presently being followed, and the two children most recently shunted for hydrocephalus show normal intellectual functioning and no evidence of psychomotor delay at the age of two years. The remaining eight children have signs of cerebral palsy ranging from mild to severe, although only one child demonstrates intellectual functioning within the retarded range, and one infant with severe spastic quadriplegia demonstrates an intelligence quotient within the superior range.

Presently, 67 children of multiple births who were hospitalized in the intensive care unit are being followed. Of these, 15 children are handicapped, yielding a 22-percent handicapping incidence. The breakdown of handicapping conditions is as follows: cerebral palsy, eight; hearing-handicapped cerebral palsy, one; cerebral palsy with mental retardation, one; mental retardation, two; hearing handicap, two; blindness and mental retardation, one.

Throughout all diagnostic groups, cerebral palsy is the most frequently observed neurological sequela of prematurity and neonatal asphyxia. While the psychomotor delay is accompanied initially by mental scores within the retarded range, these scores generally improve with verbal functioning, so that the I.Q. for these physically handicapped children improves with age, and several are within the superior to gifted ranges.

There are many clinical uses of the developmental follow-up evaluation of the neonatal intensive care unit survivor. Results of the evaluation can provide reassurance to the parents as well as identification of significant delays. Appropriate avenues for remediation are often indicated through testing. The process of the evaluation itself provides opportunities for teaching parents about normal developmental behaviors and expectations and provides parents with a better understanding of their infant's own temperament and learning style.

Timing for longitudinal evaluations is crucial and depends upon the needs of the parents and infants as well as the questions being asked by the examiner. The psychologist with a strong background in child development is in a position to assess overall psychological functioning and to refer to specialized assessments (i.e., speech and language or occupational therapy) if a multidisciplinary team is not available on site.

There are important considerations in testing infants, which include separation, the importance of the family unit, physical setting, and timing. Providing feedback to parents is the most critical aspect of infant testing and requires careful consideration of the needs of the parents.

REFERENCES

Als, H., Tronick, E., Adamson, L., and Brazelton, T. The behavior of the full-term but underweight newborn infant. *Developmental Medicine and Child Neurology, 18,* 590-602 (1976).

Black, L., Steinscheider, A., and Sheehe, P.R. Neonatal respiratory instability and infant development. *Child Development, 50,* 561–564 (1979).

Cronback, L.J. *Essentials of Psychological Testing,* 2nd ed. Harper & Bros., New York (1960).

Drillien, C.M. *The Growth and Development of the Prematurely Born Infant.* Livingstone, Edinburgh (1964).

Field, T.M., Sostek, A.M., Goldberg, S., and Shuman, H.H., eds. *Infants Born At Risk,* Spectrum, New York (1979).

Huntington, D.S. Supportive programs for infants and parents. In *Handbook of Infant Development,* J.D. Osofsky, ed. Wiley, New York (1979), pp. 837–851.

Luick, A., and Williams, E.. Factors affecting interpretation of psychological tests. *The Newborn Follow-Up, 3,* No. 6 (1979) [an internal newsletter of the University of Arizona Health Sciences Center, Department of Pediatrics, Section of Neonatal Biology].

McDonald, A.D. Intelligence in children of very low birth weight. *British Journal of Preventive and Social Medicine, 18,* 59–74 (1964).

Mercer, H.P., Lancaster, P.A.L., Weiner, T., and Gupta, J.M. Very low birth-weight infants. *Medical Journal of Australia, 2,* 581–584 (1978).

Osofsky, J., ed. *Handbook of Infant Development.* Wiley, New York (1979), p. 51.

Parmelee, A.H., and Schulte, F. Developmental testing of pre-term and small-for-dates infants. *Pediatrics, 45,* 21–28 (1970).

Saint-Anne Dargassies, S. Neurological maturation of the premature infant of 28 to 40 weeks' gestational age. In *Human Development,* F. Falkner, ed. W.B. Saunders, Philadelphia (1966).

–––. Long-term neurolological follow-up study of 286 truly premature infants. I: Neurological sequelae. *Developmental Medicine and Child Neurology, 19,* 462–478 (1977).

Scott, H. Outcome of very severe birth asphyxia. *Archives of Disease in Childhood, 51,* 712 (1976).

Solomons, G. Child abuse and developmental disabilities. *Devepmental Medicine and Child Neurology, 21,* 101–108 (1979).

Stewart, A.L., Turcan, D.M., Rawlings, G., and Reynolds, E.O.R. Prognosis for infants weighing 1000 g or less at birth. *Archives of Disease in Childhood, 52,* 97–104 (1977).

Teberg, A., Hodgman, J.E., Wu, P.Y.K., and Spears, R.L. Recent improvement in outcome for the small premature infant. *Clinical Pediatrics, 16,* 307–313 (1977).

7

The Role of a Psychologist in a Pediatric Setting

Jack Wetter

The purpose of this chapter is to provide a summary review of the behavioral and psychological aspects of pediatrics.

Psychology as a science appeared relatively late: well after anatomy, physiology, chemistry, and physics. Psychology is to be looked on as the science that concerns itself with the main trends or general laws that guide and control the behavior of human beings in relationship to their physical environment and to one another.

In a sense, every individual in the world is a practical psychologist because he is engaged in the process of adjusting himself, of meeting other people and of reacting to them, and because, whether he likes it or not, he must formulate principles of conduct and deductions with reference to the conduct of others.

Early in the development of a collaborative liaison between psychology and pediatrics, there was evidence of a distinction between psychology as a systematized body of knowledge about human development and the practice of psychology within a medical setting. The first perspective taken, over 40 years ago, separated the clinical functions of psychology from the scientific or didactic functions (Anderson, 1930). Essentially, Anderson contended that psychology contributed two major insights toward the understanding and care of the sick child: the tools to better assess cognitive capacities and a body of empirically derived knowledge about the development and training of young children. To the extent that psychologists are viewed as expert consultants in behavioral science, their role vis-à-vis pediatric practice remains essentially as Anderson described it.

Further elaboration of this role was provided by Kagan (1965), who places emphasis on the research and applied theory aspects of psychology and views the liaison as mutually beneficial. The pediatrician, he points out, has much to gain from an exposure to the theoretical and research underpinnings of psychology. He goes on to postulate that as a result of collaboration, both psychologists and pediatricians develop a mental set that allows them to approach problems of child behavior and personality development from a multifaceted perspective.

In addition, each discipline acquires research skills from the other. This, he contends, is the content of a "new marriage" between psychology and pediatrics.

Schofield (1969) describes the evolution of the "medical psychologist" as a practitioner who utilizes the same scientist-clinician skills as his better-known clinical psychologist counterpart. In examining the scientist-clinician role, Wright (1967) has suggested that the role, and hence the functions, of the pediatric psychologist evolve from his training in both clinical and developmental psychology. However, Salk (1970) takes different perspective and considers the primary function of the pediatric psychologist as a specialist or resource consultant. Salk takes pains to emphasize that the pediatric psychologist is immediately available and able to provide the pediatrician with information that would facilitate appropriate and rapid dispositions.

Similar observations have been made by Smith, Rowe, and Friedheim (1967). They note that the role of the psychologist in the pediatrician's office is that of the "specialist consultant" and requires input in the area of child development, learning problems, and study habits. The authors suggested that placing a psychologist in the pediatrician's office produced two important changes: (1) a reduction of the waiting period for an appointment with the psychologist and (2) an increase in the effectiveness of communication between psychologist and pediatrician.

King, Anderson and Wiens (1972) have described the pediatric psychologist's functions in terms of child diagnostician, parent counselor, community resource, and pediatrician's consultant. In their view, training in the areas of child development and clinical child psychology are essential but not sufficient elements in the repertoire of a pediatric psychologist. It seems that there is little, if any, consensus as to precisely what skills a pediatric psychologist should possess and even less consensus as to the professional functions he might pursue. Thus, it appeared reasonable, at this juncture, to seek a statement of the pediatrician's needs as a consumer of the pediatric psychologist's service.

Stabler and Murray (1973) state that if a new role-set for psychology in pediatrics is to be established, there are two antecedent conditions that must be met. First, the emphasis on psychometrics must be placed in proper perspective with regard to the diagnosis and treatment of children. Often diagnosis involves a great deal more than the administration and evaluation of tests. By emphasizing and enhancing the longitudinal nature of psychodiagnosis, the psychologist both educates his pediatric colleagues and better serves his patients. Second, it is incumbent upon the pediatric psychologist to use his consultative skills to facilitate the communication between all disciplines operating in the pediatric setting. One way in which this may come about is through continuing in-service education programs in which the psychologist functions as a resource person and a teacher.

Although formerly neglected, the role of behavioral medicine and health care psychology for children is rapidly expanding. We live in a time when over half of all visits to medical doctors concern problems of nonorganic origin. This, of course, is making physicians more mindful of the emotional and psychological aspects of the problems they are called upon to treat. At the same time, psychologists, psychiatrists, and other behavioral practitioners, including physicians, are discovering the vast amount of psychopathology related to organic illness.

Psychosomatic illness generally connotes a physical problem, such as an ulcer, hives, or asthma, caused by emotional stress. Diabetes and hemophilia are two diseases that can indirectly produce disturbances of affect and personality. A child with diabetes often manifests passive self-destructiveness by not obtaining urine samples or taking insulin and by a general sense of apathy. Hemophilia patients often take inexplicable risks, such as riding recklessly on a motorcycle or running barefoot over hazardous ground. Such behavior is inadvisable for any young child, but it is particularly unwise for a hemophiliac. The behavior might be the result of a counterphobic reaction to anxiety or may be motivated by anger aimed at parents who are vulnerable to such expressions because of guilt from having genetically caused the disease. The point here is that these emotional problems are caused by illness and not vice versa, as is usual with typical psychosomatic problems.

There are also problems of behavior and development that result directly from diseases and through clearly understood mechanisms. Examples include burns and disfigurements, which appear to leave not only the children but their parents emotionally scarred, and Rocky Mountain spotted fever, which is known to affect both abstract thinking and perceptual-motor skills.

Sophistication in understanding and treating problems like these has increased greatly in recent years through collaborative efforts involving pediatricians and psychologists.

By 1960, pediatrics in the United States had entered a new era. There was a general leveling off of the gains in the battle against infant and child mortality and morbidity. With the general shift of the population from small towns to urban and suburban areas, the pediatrician was called upon more and more to give child-rearing advice previously available from aunts, grandmothers, and close neighbors. The popular books of Gesell and Spock also contributed to the professionalization of advice about child rearing. Responding to these new demands being made on the pediatrician, Wilson (1964), in a presidential address to the American Pediatric Society, asked the question: "Who is to attend to the common emotional or behavioral problems of children?" Wilson thought that psychologists were part of the answer.

Wright (1967) defined a pediatric psychologist as "any psychologist who finds himself dealing primarily with children in a medical setting which is nonpsychiatric in nature." In discussing the training of such a professional, Wright stated, "Ideally the pediatric psychologist is a person who is competently trained in both child development and in the child clinical area."

Pediatric psychology has developed since 1968 into self-awareness as a field in which professional psychologists work with children in nonpsychiatric medical settings such as children's hospitals, developmental clinics, and pediatric offices.

Wright (1967) further writes that over one-half of all the psychopathology of children in this world is related to a physical-behavioral symptom of some sort, for which help is usually sought first from a pediatrician or other medical doctor, and that less than one-half of the psychopathology of children falls within the traditional nosological categories of neurosis, psychosis, and character disorder.

Ideally the pediatric psychologist is a person who is competently trained in both child development and in the child clinical area. Knowledge of child development and in the child clinical area. Knowledge of child development is an essential part of the understanding necessary in the performance of psychological work, as well as a vital ingredient in making the psychologist a valuable teacher and consultant who aids medical colleagues and students in their respective endeavors. Training in the clinical area is, of course, necessary if the psychologist is to be a contributing member of a medical treatment or teaching team.

Requests for developmental and/or cognitive appraisals are disproportionately high by comparison to the requirements of a psychiatric setting. For this reason, the pediatric psychologist should be predisposed toward and uniquely skilled in making such evaluations.

In addition to possessing an unusual knowledge concerning child development, cognitive appraisals, and normal personality, the pediatric psychologist might best contribute to the effectiveness of patient care if he possess two additional predispositions: toward economy and toward the applied. The pediatrician and, for the most part, the entire pediatric setting is not geared to treatment that involves extensive amounts of professional time being expended with single patients. Time is more limited, and volume is higher. Cases cannot be handled by such techniques as long-term individual psychotherapy. Since the psychodiagnostic and, particularly, the psychotherapeutic areas of the mental field are in dire need of methods that are more economical, it seems reasonable that pediatric psychology might focus upon research designed to uncover methods that are temporally and financially efficient.

In a survey of pediatricians' perceptions of pediatric psychologists, it was found that often physicians stereotype the role of psychologists in the medical setting (Stabler and Murray, 1973). The results of this survey suggested that physicians have a tendency to circumscribe the role functions of the psychologist and to emphasize only the testing and diagnostic functions. This view, it could be argued, is at least in part the result of years of attitudinal development in the medical sciences toward the behavioral sciences. If psychologists are ever to break away from this stereotype, they must be responsible for taking the initiative to broaden their physician colleagues' view and understanding of the function of psychologists. Thus, more sophisticated and interactive models of consultation-liaison are called for.

Stabler (1973) described a useful "process consultation model." In such an interaction, it might be expected that the psychologist would have some contact with the patient, perhaps in a diagnostic testing or interview session, and would then transmit and interpret those data through a dialogue with the primary care physician consultee. This interaction provides a vehicle for the transmission of developmental and psychological information, data relevant to psychometric or projective test results and findings, opportunities for the psychologist to model the technical skills of patient interviewing and assessment, and finally, it would provide a framework within which the physician consultee could begin to learn some aspects of community consultation. This is a model often used in many pediatric psychiatry liaison programs, where the primary emphasis is on training and education of pediatric residents and medical students. However, although psychologists are generally eager to become involved in this kind of endeavor, they are often very poorly equipped in terms of their formal training in consultation-liaison approaches (Rhodes, 1974).

As an example of the specific role that a pediatric psychologist provides, one can present the following case presentation:

> Judy, a 16-year-old high school student, has for the past nine months experienced intermittent headaches associated with dizziness and nausea. This caused her to miss as much as 35 days of school in the past year. She was hospitalized two times for complete neurological and laboratory examinations. Although she was evaluated by three different physicians, no physiological cause for her symptoms was determined. Finally, in desperation, her parents brought her to a large university teaching hospital to be seen by a pediatric neurologist. A psychological consultation was requested.
>
> The pediatric resident managing Judy's case called for psychological consultation with some reluctance, believing that the symptoms represented nothing more than an attempt to avoid going to school. He felt that Judy would profit from a talk about what her "real" problem is. However, the social worker collaborating with the psychologist discovered that Judy's mother died one year previously of brain cancer. Judy's complaints closely resembled those of her mother. The psychologist and social worker, after discussing the case with the resident, gained the impression that Judy is a youngster who is out of touch with many of her emotions,

using the defense mechanisms of repression and denial as her means of coping.

Schofield (1969) has suggested that in the future psychologists who work in health maintenance organizations (HMOs) will have, in addition to their traditional clinical and research roles, the role of an educational consultant to the health care team. In this role, a psychologist would have the opportunity to contribute to general staff training with a view toward facilitating the integration of comprehensive health care to the patient. Stabler (1973) defends this process by what he terms a "Process-Educative Consultation Model." This approach does not necessarily call for the psychologist to have direct contact with the patient. In point of fact, it is often more useful that the consulting psychologist deal mainly with the impressions and perceptions of the patient as offered by the physician consultee rather than with his or her own clinical judgments.

To return to the case of Judy for a moment, we can see how this type of liaison between psychologist and pediatrician might unfold. Later, these data are discussed in a joint conference with a social worker, psychologist, pediatric attending, and the resident. The pediatric resident, although still questioning the authenticity of Judy's symptoms, is able to acknowledge a strong psychological component to the case. It is jointly decided that the best approach for the moment is to offer Judy the support necessary for her to return to school. This is accomplished through the resident contacting the school counselor and enlisting his aid and understanding, clarifying the medical-psychological picture for Judy's local physician, and giving the reassurance to Judy and her family that although her headache pain is "real," there is no physical cause for it. The resident is supported, in turn, by the consulting psychologist as he follows Judy in weekly clinic visits for a checkup and a few minutes of talking together. Although no "cure" for Judy is found, there is no doubt that her symptoms begin to diminish and are less troublesome as this relationship develops over the remainder of the school year.

A physician responsible for Judy's management would, through this type of consultation-liaison teaching, entertain not only biomedical possibilities, but would also be sensitive to and aware of the many psychosocial components operating in the case. The net result would be that the patient would receive the highest level of health care available to her. This position can be reached only when medical and behavioral specialists are able to adequately and efficiently communicate with each other; when, in other words, the process of consultation-liaison comes full circle.

Today, perhaps as never before, the pediatrician more than any other professional holds a most influential role for the mental health of future generations. Only recently has it become known how profound the effects of early experience on later behavior can be.

The pediatrician sees more human beings during their most critical phases of development than any other professional person. Often he detects developmental and psychological problems and is in a position to recommend further study of the problems and methods for dealing with them, or to refer to another professional for treatment.

The pediatrician is looked upon as an expert in child-rearing practices, but, more often than not, lacks the knowledge and training required for such a role. Part of the reason for this gap in pediatric training lies in the fact that medical centers rely on psychiatry for training in human behavior rather than on the broader behavioral sciences that focus more on psychological theory and social organization. Traditionally, it has been the psychiatrist to whom the pediatrician was expected to turn for his knowledge of human behavior, and very often the problems the pediatrician is concerned with do not require the traditional psychiatric approach, but require a broader knowledge of psychological theory.

Clearly, pediatricians must receive more intensive training in the behavioral sciences, particularly in personality growth and development. Furthermore, the pediatrician should have available a consultant trained in the behavioral sciences and equipped to screen, diagnose, and advise on problems pertaining to development, learning, behavior disorders, nervous dysfunction, and patient management, as well as child-rearing practices. This psychological consultant should be available to pediatricians without delay, so that they can continue to assume responsibility for their patients without loss of continuity, can become more sensitized to psychological factors, and be more adept in "feeling out" potential problems. By working closely with such a consultant, pediatricians will be able to deal with patients medically without loss of time or unnecessary involvement, while offering good mental health service. What is fast becoming a new specialty in psychology—pediatric psychology—has grown out of the need on the part of the pediatrician for such a consultant.

The pediatric psychologist, like the clinical child psychologist, has the basic concerns of prevention and treatment of behavior disorders of children. He stresses the philosophy of expedient methods of assessment and crisis treatment with an acute regard for the goal of prevention.

The pediatric psychologist who works in pediatric settings is available to the pediatrician upon short notice to answer questions regarding psychological matters, and he works directly with the pediatric staff as a consultant (Salk, 1974).

In practice, the pediatric psychologist is called upon to help pediatricians understand normal psychological growth and development; to help counsel parents about child-rearing issues; and to recognize and, where possible, remediate disorders of development. Diagnostic services of the pediatric psychologist also involve developmental or intellectual appraisal determined by specialized techniques not usually found in the clinical child psychologist's practice.

The pediatric setting is not geared to treatment requiring long-term involvement. The request for psychological consultation is quickly dealt with by providing immediate consultation. Efficiency is necessary for three tasks: (1) immediate screening to eliminate delays for necessary disposition; (2) early diagnosis of learning, developmental, and emotional problems; and (3) communication of the formulation of the case based upon psychological principles to the pediatric staff.

The concepts of minimal brain damage, dyslexia, hyperkinetic behavior disorders, special learning problems, and psychosomatic disorders have emphasized the interrelationship between physical and psychological development. Thus, medical programs have become dependent upon this dimension of psychological understanding and support, and psychologists active in schools and medical clinics have had increased contact with medical problems. This has emphasized the need for the psychologist to be trained in all aspects of normal child development as well as in specific developmental disabilities. The pediatric psychologist has evolved to diagnose and to counsel children in a medical setting that is essentially nonpsychiatric.

The trainee in pediatric psychology deals with an age spectrum ranging from infancy through adolescence and with multiple problems, including mental retardation, learning disabilities, speech and language problems, as well as physical and developmental disorders that have psychological and emotional components.

Both clinical child psychology and pediatric psychology have in common concerns with the theoretical aspects of behavior and development of the child population. They are both, in addition, clinical psychology specialties. The differentiating features are the locus of professional activities as well as the specific aspects of behaviors of the target population. The clinical child psychologist most typically practices in a psychiatrically oriented setting, a medical school, a mental health center, or a clinic, whereas the pediatric psychologist practices in a pediatric department of a hospital, medical school, or private-practice setting. The target population of the clinical child psychologist is most typically designated by his immediate environment as being behaviorally deviant. The child of concern to the pediatric psychologist is more likely to be suffering from the rapid onset of behavioral deviations precipitated by medical or hospital procedures or a physical illness.

With the increased recognition of pediatric psychology as a subspecialty, it can be hoped that we are at the end of the era in which the child's total development was ignored in medical settings, and the many behavioral concomitants of physical illness were ignored. We begin an era in which pediatric psychologists, as well as the many other behavioral practitioners, are better prepared to respond to the variety of psychiatric, psychosomatic, developmental, learning, and other illness-related problems that are encountered in children's medical settings. Many disorders such as enuresis, encopresis, psychogenic vomiting, and an array of previously baffling conditions are now being treated with a high degree of success by pediatric psychologists.

REFERENCES

Anderson, J.A. Pediatrics and child psychology. *Journal of the American Medical Association, 95,* 1015-1018 (1930).

Kagan, J. The new marriage: Pediatrics and psychology. *American Journal of Diseases of Childhood, 110,* 272-278 (1975).

King, H.E., Anderson, K.A., and Wiens, A.N. A pediatric psychology residency program. Unpublished manuscript, University of Oregon, Eugene (1972).

Rhodes, W.C. Principles and practices of consultation. *Professional Psychology, 27,* 587-589 (1974).

Salk, L. Psychologist in a pediatric setting. *Professional Psychology, 1,* 395-396 (1970).

———. Psychologist and pediatrician: A mental health team in the prevention and early diagnosis of mental disorders. In *Clinical Child Psychology: Current Practices and Future Perspectives,* G.J. Williams and S. Gordon, eds. Behavioral Publications, New York (1974), pp. 110-115.

Schofield, W. The role of psychology in the delivery of health services. *American Psychologist, 24,* 565-584 (1969).

Smith, E.E., Rowe, L.P., and Freedheim, D.K. The clinical psychologist in the pediatric office. *Journal of Pediatrics, 71,* 48-51 (1967).

Stabler, B., and Murray, J.P. Pediatricians' perceptions of pediatric psychology. *Clinical Psychologist, 27,* 12-15 (1973).

Wilson, J.L. Growth and development of pediatrics. *Journal of Pediatrics, 65,* 984-991 (1964).

Wright, L. The pediatric psychologist: A role model. *American Psychologist, 22,* 323-325 (1967).

8

Cognitive Skills and the Learning-disabled Youngster

Nita Ferjo

INTRODUCTION

The business of children is to go to school. Six hours a day, five days a week, ten to twenty years of their lives children and adolescents are involved in acquiring formal education. Schools are the only mandatory program for children. No law requires that children see a pediatrician, live with relatives, or attend religious services, yet they *must* be involved in an educational program (Ely, 1980, *California Laws Relating to Minors*).

The rules of school attendance are well defined. The space allotted, credentials of staff, age restrictions for students, subjects taught, texts used, etc., are all carefully planned. Six-year-olds are in kindergarten or first grade. By the time the majority of regular students reach their 18th birthday, graduation from high school is imminent. Placement in a grade at school is determined by chronological age—not by physical size, specific skills or the lack thereof, but rather by the fate of birth date. Speaking English isn't even a requirement; rather, the school asks for the child's birth certificate to determine registration in a class. No child is retained indefinitely in one grade of school, but progresses up through the system to obtain a high school certificate after 12th grade. From that point onward, education is optional.

EDUCATIONAL CONTINGENCIES

When one considers what is required of children to survive and succeed in school, it is amazing that it is accomplished at all! The average grade in the average school in the United States, whether it be Maine, Louisiana, or California, consists of 20 to 35 students within a three-year age range, in a room with one teacher. Each child is assigned a seat, texts, and a series of assignments. The teacher gives the instructions by talking or writing. Then, the child's response in writing or speaking is evaluated according to correctness within a certain time frame. The student must attend, comprehend the instructions, and block out distractions and stimuli within the room while focusing on accomplishing the assigned tasks. Simultaneously, the student must be sensitive to the numerous behavioral rules for that classroom, which may include seat sitting, hand raising, paper folding, or ignoring noisy friends. A child must learn the numerous social rules of the school scene. One can yell and run in the playground, but not in the class room. Conduct in the principal's office is different from that in the cafeteria or with peers. The social milieu and academic demands become extremely complex; yet the majority of children successfully master each stage and progress through the system to become literate, educated, socialized adults.

ELEMENTS OF READING

In addition to socializing children and teaching them to work in groups, the business of school is to teach children how to do reading, writing, spelling, and mathematics. The primary focus in the primary grades is on reading, since all future education still depends upon the child's ability to get information from the written page. (This focus may be rapidly changing with television and the electronic age.)

When one analyzes the components of reading, one realizes that it is a highly complex skill, which requires a high degree of discrimination, memory, organization, and an acceptance of the nonsensical.

First, the student must learn over 100 symbols (Fig. 8-1). These symbols have little or no logical explanation for their formation. P,p, follows a progression. So does M,m, with some variation, but how does a child or teacher explain B,b, R,r, or D,d. The child must simply memorize these facts.

Aa Bb Cc Dd Ee Ff Gg Hh Ii Jj Kk Ll Mm Nn Oo Pp Qq Rr Ss Tt Uu Vv
Ww Xx Yy Zz , . : ; " ' / ? ! # $ % ¢ & * ( ) — - + = ÷ > < □ △ ○ 0 1 2 3 4
5 6 7 8 9

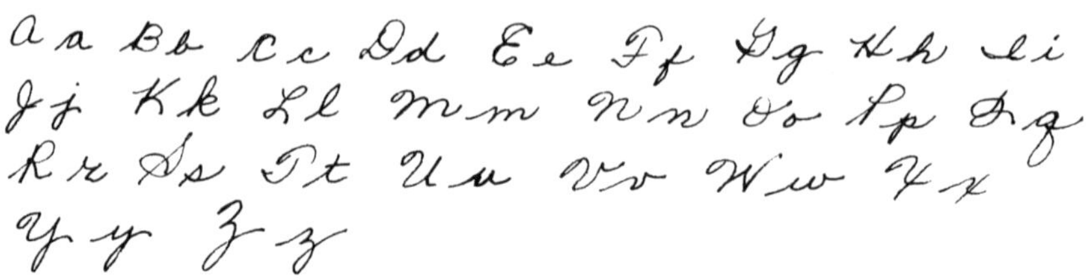

Figure 8-1

Not only must the student memorize the symbols, but these letters must be clustered together to form words, with spaces in between, which provide critical units of information. Meaning changes as letters are added, deleted, or arranged in a different order.

Example:
I have a red book.
I have read a book.

Simultaneously, the youngster must attach auditory sounds to those non-descript symbols. No sooner are the consonants learned, with all of the exceptions (*K* and *C* sound alike in *car* and *kite*; *C* and *S* sound alike in *send* and *cent*; but forget the next step in logical reasoning, because *S* and *K* rarely if ever sound alike), then the vowels are introduced, with the numerous minor inflections. If one has frequent hearing losses due to colds and congestions, a foreign accent, or a short-term auditory memory, this may be a very difficult area of learning.

Additionally, since English was derived from a conglomerate of other languages, it is riddled with silent letters in spelling plus identical pronunciations for two words that are spelled differently:

Example:
site   sight
write   right
know   no

Not only must a child remember the visual symbols and auditory correlates, but, in addition to correct verbalization and comprehension, reproduction on the page is expected. The youngster who writes English must begin at the left border of the page and move horizontally across on the line, dropping down to the next line at proper intervals between or within words to continue the process (Japanese and Hebrew require different spatial organization).

If the student masters the rules for copying words and sentences, mathematics introduces new complications, and the rules for organization on the page change.

Example:
$7 + 3 =$ is the same as $3 + 7 =$
but
$7 - 3 =$ is not the same as $3 - 7 =$

The distinctions are subtle but critical in the computations, and the spatial organization is a critical variable when determining the process and correct answer.

If a child has a weakness in the ability to comprehend, organize, retain, recall, and synthesize the numerous segments of the highly technical skills required in each of the facets of reading and arithmetic (but more often in reading), then failure in the primary business of education occurs.

That youngster becomes a frustration to parents, teachers, and the school system. The child is initially identified as failing, and may be accused of being unmotivated, uncooperative, not working up to potential; or worse yet—a slow learner, learning disabled, or retarded.

The family seeks assistance from professionals, often going first to the family doctor, hoping there is a physical reason for this problem. This author does not pretend to tell the physician how to do a physical examination of a learning-disabled child, even though there is a higher incidence of soft neurological signs and physically abnormal presentations among these students, but this is where it should begin (Kinsbourne and Caplan, 1979; Wender, 1971).

INCIDENCE OF EXCEPTIONALITY

Two to twenty percent of the school population (Hewitt and Forness, 1977, p. 76), depending on the source of the statistics and the groups identified as exceptional, cannot function in a regular classroom without assistance and intervention. Because of this, special education was developed. Historically, handicapped children were segregated from the normal population. Schools for the deaf, blind, physically handicapped, and retarded were developed. This did not account for yet another group, which remained in the classrooms—the youngsters with behavioral, emotional, speech, and academic problems. Their disabilities were more subtle, less easily defined, and could not be attributed to some obvious physical deficit.

EDUCATIONAL CLASSES

It was comfortable to follow the medical model when placing students in special schools and classes because of some known physical deficit, such as cerebral palsy, down's syndrome, or deafness, even though there was much disparity between their academic skills that did not relate to the physical complaints. How was the new subgroup that still was not progressing in the regular classroom to be defined? Educators developed classes for the mildly retarded, language delayed, and educationally disabled, always focusing on the deficit as the reason for placement in special programs (Sapir and Wilson, 1978). Parents and educators became unhappy with the inequities and isolation that these students were experiencing, and began pushing for change.

NEW DIRECTIONS IN EDUCATION

The enactment of the Education for All Handicapped Children Act (Public Law 94-142) in 1975 has far-reaching and profound implications for how special students are viewed, assessed, and served in the educational system. It stipulates that all handicapped children must have a free and appropriate education in the least restrictive environment, with related services available as needed. The law assures that federal monies will be provided to the states so that all children, ages 3 to 21, who are assessed as needing special services can be provided with an appropriate education.

Public Law (PL) 94-142 designates the procedures by which a child is to be assessed so that the testing is nondiscriminatory. The parents are entitled to all school records, prior notice of school actions regarding their child, and an impartial hearing if they are not satisfied with any segment of the assessment or services provided to their child. The cornerstone of PL 94-142 is its provision for a written, individualized educational plan for each child. This individual educational plan (IEP) is to include the child's present level of functioning, goals and objectives, the services to be provided and time allotted each service, a starting date, and expected duration. The IEP must be reviewed on at least a yearly basis, and a parent can initiate a review at any time, with due process and a fair hearing provided (Hewett and Forness, 1977, p. 568). These categories now evaluate the child's strengths, as well as weaknesses, stressing normalization and mainstreaming of youngsters back into the regular classroom, with support services.

LEARNING DISABILITIES

Public Law 94-142 is not just a law for the physically disabled or retarded. Funds are also allotted for the learning-disabled student. What is a specific learning disability?

The National Committee on Handicapped Children currently defines it as follows:

> 'Specific learning disability' means a disorder in one or more of the basic psychological processes involved in understanding or in using language, spoken or written, which may manifest itself in an imperfect ability to listen, think, speak, read, write, spell or do mathematical calculations. The term includes such conditions as perceptual handicaps, brain injury, minimal brain dysfunction, dyslexia and developmental aphasia. The term does not include children who have learning problems which are primarily the result of visual, hearing, or motor handicaps, of mental retardation or emotional disturbance, or of environmental, cultural, or economic disadvantage. (USOE, 1977, p. 65083)

Because the rules of PL 94-142 mandate a nondiscriminatory assessment by a team to determine the child's area of strengths and weaknesses, it is necessary to rule out the myriad of other factors before a child is considered as having a primary learning disability.

Assessment

The evaluation of the special education student is meant to be a group effort, with input from the family, teacher, physicians, and school professionals. All of this is done with full permission and knowledge of the parents. The student, where advisable, is also given the right of choice plus feedback regarding the procedures and findings. Parents can request an assessment of their child by the school district psychologist.

A thorough assessment should include the following:

1. Physical examination
2. Developmental and educational history
3. Behavioral ratings and observations
4. Academic testing
5. Cognitive assessment
6. Perceptual testing
7. Speech and language evaluation
8. Description of social-emotional status

Some school districts would group together all of the testing except the physical examination into what is called a psychoeducational evaluation (Sapir and Wilson, 1978, p. 7). Included would be information on the intellectual, perceptual (visual, auditory, motoric, and integrative abilities), language, and emotional development, as well as educational skills.

Physical Examination

A careful physical examination is the first level of assessment and is a critical component in the assessment of children who are not progressing in school. The physical examination should include: (1) vision, (2) hearing, and (3) a neurological examination. A child with a mild visual problem often does not know that he/she doesn't see as well as the next child, and may be mislabeled as a child with visual-perceptual difficulty, rather than a youngster with true visual problems, which could readily be corrected.

Additionally, youngsters with mild or intermittent hearing losses due to allergies or upper respiratory infections get labeled by the teacher as inattentive, or lower functioning if the problem goes undetected. A first grader with chronic lowered hearing is particularly at risk for failure when a teacher utilizes a phonetic approach to reading.

Kinsbourne and Caplan make a strong case for a thorough physical exam, stating:

> A variety of diseases can produce school failure as one of their symptoms and occasionally confusion with learning disability is possible. Anemia, malnutrition, parasite infestation, and other debilitating conditions can make a child listless in the classroom. . . . In rare cases a child progressively loses ground in school as an early symptom of a progressive brain degeneration. One rare simulator of chronic inattentiveness is the epileptic variant, status petit mal that produces momentary lapses of consciousness (Kinsbourne and Caplan, 1979, pp. 92-93).

According to these authors, a routine neurological examination of learning-disabled children often shows a variety of minor physical signs indicating abnormality or immaturity of the central nervous system.

It can be argued that these youngsters have deficits, are just immature, or are structurally different from their peers. The theorizing lends little assistance to the educational program for the child. These minor neurological findings often have profound implications in a classroom, where a student is expected not only to grasp the pencil correctly, but to use it as a finely tuned instrument to place small legible figures on short narrow lines in a process known as writing.

Additionally, the child is expected to participate in group games in the playground, which requires coordination, agility, and speed. The clumsy child with "soft" neurological signs is at risk for being ostracised or teased by peers when unable to compete in the physical play.

These children are at high risk to be identified and labeled as learning disabled. At risk also is their emotional development as they view themselves as different and failing.

Another role of the physician is to rule out or confirm the presence of hyperactivity or attentional deficit disorder and then monitor the medication as indicated (Cantwell, 1975; Kinsbourne and Caplan, 1979; Wender, 1971). Hyperactivity and its impact in the school setting as a major factor in causing the youngster to function poorly are well documented.

Developmental and Educational History

Parents are sometimes reluctant to give detailed birth histories to the school; yet, it is critical to the understanding of the child's present functioning to understand whether all of the developmental milestones were delayed or whether there was a recent difficulty. Researchers are now beginning to tie early histories of language delay to later dyslexia. It is also suggested that certain types of learning problems run in families and may have a genetic basis.

A careful school history is essential to determine whether the child has had adequate exposure to appropriate educational programs. Chronically ill, migrant, and phobic children often miss critical training periods, which can guarantee school failure if appropriate remediation is not provided.

A language history is also important—not only the rate of acquisition of language, but what was the predominant language in the child's preschool years. Further research in this area may focus on the acquisition of language, or the lack thereof, as having long-term educational effects, rather than the present preoccupation with 'soft' neurological signs.

Behavioral Ratings and Observations

Because standardized testing can only evaluate a small segment of behavior in a prescribed manner and time, it is important to attempt to develop the larger picture of the child in his environment. First, one needs some indication of the bias of the observers and what are their criteria for normalcy.

Smith states: "It is important to remember that the value of the information collected depends on how reliably and validly it characterizes the typical, usual behavior of the youngsters under observation. It is the child's normal behavior that must be of concern to the teacher" (Smith, 1969, p. 213). Reliability of observations can be increased by observing in various settings and by reassessing over time.

Often a physician or the school personnel will attempt to get more formalized data by utilizing scales that compare the target student to other normal children within the classroom. Examples of such scales are:

1. *Devereux Elementary School Behavior Rating Scale* (Spivack and Swift, 1967). This contains 47 items that are rated on a seven-point scale to yield composite scores on 11 subscales, which give information about items such as classroom disturbance, achievement, anxiety, and inattentiveness.
2. *Conners Teacher Questionnaire* (Conners, 1969). This questionnaire looks at the behavior of possibly hyperactive youngsters.
3. *Pupil Rating Scale: Screening for Learning Disabilities* (Myklebust, 1971). This scale asks teachers to rate youngsters in five areas where they may present with difficulty in school, including hearing, spoken language, orientation, coordination, and behavior.

Numerous other scales have been developed to look at the behavior of particular groups (Quay, 1977) and may better describe the child in relationship to the subculture from which he/she may come.

Academic Testing

Since failure in school is determined in either behavioral or academic terms, ongoing daily testing and assessment of the child's functioning in the class must become part of the total evaluation of the student. The role of the examiner is to determine what skills the child has acquired and under what conditions. Some children need additional time but understand all concepts. Others may be able to verbalize answers but have far more difficulty writing the information down on paper. Some cannot function in the hustle and bustle of a stimulating class-room. Specific strengths and deficits are common problems of the learning-disabled child. Achievement tests far too numerous to mention here have been devised by a myriad of researchers and educators.

A test that is quickly administered and is frequently used by school psychologists for screening youngsters is the *Wide Range Achievement Test* (Jastak, Bijou, and Jastak, 1978). The WRAT has three areas: reading, spelling, and arithmetic; it can be used for students from kindergarten to college, with two levels of difficulty available. It requires the student to pronounce words of increasing difficulty, but does not evaluate reading comprehension. Spelling is determined by the examiner dictating a series of words. Arithmetic consists of a page with samples of computations taught in the various grades.

Another achievement test, which analyzes more areas, is the *Peabody Individual Achievement Test* (Dunn and Markwardt, 1970). The PIAT consists of five subtests: mathematics, reading recognition, reading comprehension, spelling, and general information; it is basically a multiple-choice test, with the student being requested to choose the correct response among four, except for the general information test, where the examiner asks a question such as, "In which direction does the sun set?" and the student gives a verbal response.

Children with no learning problems will probably score in the same grade range on a series of achievement tests, but learning-disabled children have wide variability, with both inter- and intratest scatter. A child may be able to give a correct response when the cues are in front of him/her on the page, but is unable to recall from memory in spelling or math. Bright children with specific difficulty in word recall and sight vocabulary can score much better in the reading comprehension section by utilizing context clues and calculated guesses. Only a small portion of the variables need to be considered when one analyzes the task of reading and the skills required of the student.

Cognitive Assessment

To be identified as learning disabled rather than retarded, the youngster must have normal intelligence. It is a generally accepted fact that the higher the cognitive ability of the student, the greater the chance of success in academic performance. Likewise, retarded youngsters do not acquire information as rapidly as or with the fluency of normal peers. Learning-disabled children often have a scatter in their performance, so that a composite I.Q. is of little use in determining their abilities. Test scores need to be viewed with caution. Knowing a child's intelligence quotient on a test will not help the professional. As stated by Sapir and Wilson (1978, p. 14): "Children with identical IQs may have very different levels of intellectual functioning, potential, strengths and weaknesses. Also, a child who has minor illness such as a cold or who has not breakfasted or whose sleep was interrupted for any reason may test poorly. In all testing, processes are more important than products."

A variety of intelligence tests have been developed and expounded. In popular present-day use is the *Wechsler Intelligence Scale for Children, Revised* (Wechsler, 1974), developed for the school population of between 6 and 16 years of age. The test is sorted into verbal and performance items, and a full-scale score is also derived. There are 12 subtests designed to tap a variety of skills—from copying and doing puzzle-like designs to vocabulary and information. A child with a normal intelligence quotient of 100 may have a widely scattered profile, showing patterns of diversity that are highly significant when planning the educational program. The youngster with low scores in the verbal areas but high scores in the performance items is very different educationally from a child with the same I.Q. but with the reverse profile.

A second test that is frequently used is the Stanford-Binet (Terman and Merrill, 1973), which differs from the WISC-R in that it gives one score and does not have the subtests. It is more heavily weighted toward verbal cognitive skills, with few performance items.

Specialty Testing

Once a child is determined to have average intelligence and the areas of academic strengths and weaknesses are obtained, further perceptual and language testing can be utilized to explore how the student learns and what are the specific areas of strength and weakness. A variety of tests have been developed to look at eye-hand coordination, visual-motor integration, and other specific areas of learning. The testing for specific deficits is still viewed by some researchers with skepticism, and the remedial programs that evolve need to be more carefully developed. Still, it gives one more dimension of knowledge about the child who is failing in the classroom. Tests that have gained popularity are:

1. *Bender Visual Motor Gestalt Test* (Bender, 1946). This test consists of nine geometric figures, standardized for ages five and up, and requires the subject to copy the figures. By the age of 11, all children should be able to complete all designs successfully. The student's production is scored on a number of perimeters. Koppitz's (1964) text is one of the

most frequently used references for evaluating the *Bender* drawings for visual-motor errors. Emotional factors can also be scored.

2. *Developmental Test of Visual-Motor Integration* (Beery, 1967). This test is designed for ages 2½ to 15 years and asks children to copy increasingly difficult designs, arranged according to a developmental progression. It eliminates the necessity for planning and organization of space, as required by the *Bender*.

3. *The Illinois Test of Psycholinguistic Abilities* (Kirk, McCarthy, and Kirk, 1968). This test was designed with the premise that there are both representational and automatic levels of auditory-vocal and visual-motor learning. These are analyzed in 12 subtests with a series of tasks, one of which requires students to listen to sentences and determine whether they are nonsensical. Later they are to complete the sentence that the examiner initiates, such as, "A hat goes on our head, shoes go on our _____." Also, the student is shown a series of pictures and asked to determine which objects fit best with each other. The test is designed for ages 2½ to 10. It is criticized in that the subtests overlap and may be tapping learning styles and skills for which the test was not designated.

4. *Peabody Picture Vocabulary Test* (Dunn, 1965). This test, designed for ages 2½ to 18 years, is often misidentified as an intelligence test. It is a series of increasingly difficult word concepts and measures receptive language by asking the student to point to one of four pictures on the page that represents the term presented, such as "dog" and "thinking."

This brief summary does not begin to explore the myriad of tests that have been developed to assess learning-disabled students, but, rather, is designed to give only a sample of the material that can be utilized. For further information in this area, Sapir and Wilson's text, *A Professional's Guide to Working with the Learning Disabled Child* (Sapir and Wilson, 1978), gives detailed accounts of the tests, their strengths, weaknesses, and relevance to various areas of learning.

Social-Emotional Assessment

A psychoeducational evaluation by the school psychologist does not usually contain projective tests, which are dependent on the clinical skills and expertise of a professional with advanced degrees. Additionally, projective information is an interpretation of how the clinician views the child, and so is somewhat speculative. A child may give few or bizarre answers on a projective examination because of serious emotional problems, serious language problems, or receptive aphasia, making the information presented by the examiner misinterpreted or misunderstood. The responses of learning-disabled children must be viewed with caution, to rule out these factors.

Yet, the examiner needs information about how the child feels about himself/herself in relation to his/her school and peers. Much of this can be obtained through sensitive interviews with the student. Another technique is evaluation of the child's art work and drawings. Art can also be utilized to obtain information about the child's cognitive functioning. Techniques for scoring and questioning have been developed in a number of tests.

1. *Draw A Person Test* (Di Leo, 1973). The child is asked to draw himself/herself, a man, and a woman, and questions are asked about each.
2. *House-Tree-Person Test* (Buck, 1965). The youngster is requested to draw a house, a tree, and a person, and appropriate questioning follows. Family drawings can also be utilized.
3. *Secretary-Boss Test*. This examiner has developed an informal technique wherein the child who is reluctant to draw is told that he/she may be the "Boss" and can dictate or say anything they want, being encouraged to tell a story. The examiner is then the "secretary," who must write down everything said. Many children share stories of their concerns, fears, dreams; it also gives an excellent sample of daily language usage.

Individual Educational Plan (IEP)

Once the assessment is completed (utilizing information from a variety of sources, such as those described), a profile of the child, with strengths and weaknesses, can be more clearly delineated. Now the school personnel involved in the evaluation, the family, and sometimes the student (depending on age and understanding), plus all other relevant or interested persons are ready to meet so that the individual educational plan (IEP) can be written. Often parents will request advocates or outside professionals, such as the family physician, psychologist, or social worker, to attend this conference with them to more explicitly explain the needs of the student.

The IEP lists the strengths and weaknesses of the student, the primary disability, and educational goals; it specifies how these were determined and evaluated, what related services will be provided (i.e., speech therapy, physical therapy, counseling, transportation), in what setting (i.e., regular class, non-public-school placement), and how often. Additionally, a review date is stated, with one-year reviews mandated.

The IEP is where conflict may develop. Parents may or may not agree with the school's assessment. Different priorities may be presented by the family in their desire for an optimal educational program for the learning-disabled child. Often, the parents may seek services that are expensive or difficult for the school to provide, such as counseling or daily remedial physical education. Unfortunately, animosity between the school and the family may develop as the case gets prepared for a fair hearing.

Fair Hearings

If the differences cannot be settled at the IEP meeting, the parents can refuse to sign that they agree with the plan for their child. The school must advise the parents of their rights to outside assessment at school expense and to legal and advocacy services, and the date for an informal hearing within the school district is set up. If that meeting doesn't resolve the conflict, parents or school districts can take their grievances to the state level. The procedures for this are delineated in PL 94-142. During this process the child is to remain in the program in which he/she was when the negotiations were stopped, until a final resolution is made. By the time the disagreement reaches this stage, much animosity has developed on both sides. It is sometimes the role of the physician to serve as a mediator.

Determining what is "best" for the learning-disabled child is speculative, since there is no long-term research to determine who does or does not just mature out of the disability, who compensates, and who responds effectively to different types of educational intervention. Fair hearings must sometimes be based on "soft" data and clinical judgment after all the testing and assessment.

Psychological Issues

The family physician sees the child when the youngster is in pain. It is often the family who is in pain when a child fails in school. They are distraught, bewildered, unhappy. This gets communicated to the child, as well as to friends, the educational system, and the doctor. Since school is mandatory, a child who is failing in school is a failure in life. There must be a cause, or something that can be fixed. The family brings the child, looking for a physical cause. Though there may be minor anomalies or "soft" neurological signs, these don't often explain the severity of the difficulty. Other causes, such as poor teaching, unmotivated student, or absent father, are seen as reasons for the child's failure. Often there are multiple factors, and it is the interaction of these factors that tips the scale to place the child on the side of failure.

Parents in their pain may not hear, or may distort or exaggerate what the school personnel has said about the child. Parents often go through the same stages of grief, anger, and denial that are seen when they are told that their child has a terminal illness. After a visit to the physician, who tells them, "Your child is fine," the family may take that information back to the school in an accusatory fashion, blaming the school for the difficulty. As the child feels stressed, overwhelmed, and the center of conflict, his reaction ranges from hostility and belligerence to withdrawal, and even suicide in some cases. It is rare that a student with learning problems or any type of school difficulty doesn't exhibit some secondary emotional problems despite the best efforts of understanding parents and teachers.

Tact, sensitivity, and input from as many objective sources as possible can assist the physician in the role of assessing the learning-disabled child and serving as an advocate for the child with both the family and the school. The child may have no difficulty in the doctor's office, but has a specific difficulty in efficiently completing some small aspect of the highly complex and detailed tasks required in learning to read, think, speak, listen, write, and calculate. Moreover, these tasks must be performed while the child is sitting in a chair in a room filled with peers, sounds, and movement. It is fortunate that children learn at all!

REFERENCES

Beery, K.E., and Buktenica, N.A. *Developmental Test of Visual-Motor Integration.* Follett, Chicago (1967).

Bender, L., *Bender Visual Motor Gestalt Test.* American Orthopsychiatric Association (1946).

Buck, J. N. *House-Tree-Person (H-T-P) Scoring Folder.* Western Psychological Services, Los Angeles (1950).

Cantwell, D.P., ed. *The Hyperactive Child: Diagnosis, Management and Current Research.* Spectrum, New York (1975).

Conners, C.K. A teacher rating scale for use in drug studies with children. *American Journal of Psychiatry*, 884–888 (1969).

Di Leo, J.H. *Children's Drawings As Diagnostic Aids.* Brunner/Mazel, New York (1973).

Dunn, L.M. *Peabody Picture Vocabulary Test.* American Guidance Service, Circle Pines, Minn. (1965).

Dunn, L.M., and Markwardt, F.C. *Peabody Individual Achievement Test.* American Guidance Service, Circle Pines, Minn. (1965).

Ely, D.F., and Assoc., eds. *California Laws Relating to Minors.* Harcourt Brace Jovanovich, Gardena, Calif. (1980).

Hewett, F.M., and Forness, S.R. *Education of Exceptional Learners,* 2nd ed. Allyn & Bacon, Boston (1977).

Jastak, F., Bijou, S., and Jastak, S. *Wide Range Achievement Test.* Jastak Associates, Wilmington, Del. (1978).

Kinsbourne, M., and Caplan, P.J. *Children's Learning and Attentional Problems.* Little, Brown, Boston (1979).

Kirk, S.A., McCarthy, J.J., and Kirk, W.D. *Illinois Test of Psycholinguistic Abilities.* Western Psychological Services, University of Illinois Press, Urbana (1968).

Koppitz, E.M. *The Bender Gestalt Test for Young Children.* Grune & Stratton, New York (1964).

Myklebust, H.R. *The Pupil Rating Scale: Screening for Learning Disabilities.* Grune & Stratton, New York (1971).

Quay, H.C. Measuring dimensions of deviant behavior: The behavior problem checklist. *Journal of Abnormal Child Psychology, 5,* 277–289 (1977).

Sapir, S.G., and Wilson, B. *A Professional's Guide to Working with the Learning Disabled Child,* Brunner/Mazel, New York (1978).

Smith, R.M., ed. *Teacher Diagnosis of Educational Difficulties.* Charles E. Merrill, Columbus, Ohio (1969).

Spivack, G., and Swift, M. *Devereux Elementary School Behavior Rating Scale.* Devereux Foundation, Devon, Pa. (1967).

Terman, L.M., and Merrill, M.A. *Stanford-Binet Intelligence Scale.* Third Revision, Houghton Mifflin, Boston (1973).

USOE Assistance to states for education of handicapped children; procedures for evaluation of specific learning disabilities. *Federal Register, 42,* 65082–65085 (1972).

Wechsler, D. *Wechsler Intelligence Scale for Children, Revised.* The Psychological Corporation, New York (1974).

Wender, P.H. *Minimal Brain Dysfunction in Children.* Wiley-Interscience, New York (1971).

9

The Role of Psychoeducation and the
Educational Therapist in the Treatment of
Emotionally Disturbed Children

Jennifer L. Sokol

The literature of the last decade (Grace, 1974; Halpern and Kissel, 1978; Love, 1974; Schultz et al., 1973; Walsh, 1979) attests to a growing awareness and acceptance of the value and significance of the role played by the educational therapist and the psychoeducational therapist and the psychoeducational school program in the psychiatric hospital treatment of emotionally disturbed children. The purpose of this chapter is to discuss the multiple aspects of the educational therapist's role and responsibilities and to describe the manner in which the psychoeducational school program can be utilized to provide a therapeutic and growth-enhancing experience for the hospitalized child.

Ralph Colvin (1960) has stated that residential treatment of emotionally disturbed children, whether in a residential treatment center or a psychiatric hospital, represents a highly involved and many-faceted therapeutic activity for which there is no adequate preparation except past experience or the willingness to experience the new, tolerate the intolerable, and improvise the unique. Perhaps no aspect of residential treatment is more demanding of exploration, tolerance, and creative improvisation than that encountered in evolving and conducting an educational program for emotionally disturbed children. The focal significance of the educational program in residential treatment is apparent when one considers the extent to which referral for residential treatment occurs subsequent to difficulty in and often exclusion from school. Even though most school problems are related to home problems, nonetheless most often it is the school problems and the laws of compulsory education that are the immediate stimuli to hospitalization. In order to understand the role of education and the educator in the hospitalized child's treatment program, the problems typically encountered and displayed by emotionally disturbed children in public school classes prior to hospitalization will be examined.

In Western society, school is the major occupation of children and adolescents and a major focus on their attempts at adaptation and mastery. It is a social institution that is devoted to learning. It affords the child opportunities to to explore worlds previously unavailable to him/her. Within the school setting, the child can begin to utilize symbols that will permit him/her to achieve an ever increasing sense of satisfaction. Here s/he is able to relate more closely to the activities of those around him/her. S/he may now start to share more fully in a world that continues to offer one learning experience after another. For many children, this process is a pleasurable one. For the child with emotional problems, the attempts s/he makes at learning lead to conflict and dissatisfaction. His/her emotional problems are reinforced and interwoven with an inability to handle effectively the school tasks or conceptualize the school objectives.

The classroom behavior of the disturbed child is characteristically exaggerated, extreme, or stereotyped. This behavior will prevent or inhibit him/her from learning, interfere with the learning of the other students, and place undue stress on the teacher. S/he is a potential learner, but because of inflexibilities and rigidities in his/her motivation and personality, s/he is unable to learn.

The emotionally disturbed child is often unable to pursue tasks unless immediate reward or gratification is clearly visible. According to Cohen (1966), this type of child operates mainly on the pleasure principle—I want what I want when I want it. S/he cannot tolerate the slightest degree of ambiguity or abstractness in content.

Although immediate feedback is a constant necessity, the disturbed child's inability to function cuts him/her off from feedback. His/her relationship to his/her environment becomes increasingly constricted and rigid. Since s/he seems to be unable to profit from experience and has a great deal of fear and anxiety about failing, s/he is often unwilling to risk being exposed to the new, the abstract, or the symbolic. S/he often seems to expend as much energy and effort avoiding learning as the child who learns.

Knobloch (1964) pointed out that what distinguishes the disturbed child from his/her peers is not so much what s/he wants, but how s/he goes about seeking these goals and how s/he feels about the results of his/her actions. The effect of a child's emotional disturbance may distort his/her efforts at achievement and destroy their satisfying elements. Satisfaction itself may be a thing to be feared. It is the paradoxical plight of such a child that the things s/he most wish for are the things about which s/he may have the most fear.

The disturbed child not only causes and encounters difficulties in the academic aspect of the classroom, but also in his/her peer group relations. The need for peer acceptance increases as the child progresses through school. Initially, in kindergarten, his/her relationship with the teacher is needful and demanding. Rather quickly, however, the child's concern for peer group recognition becomes of prime importance. S/he strives to accomplish those things that the group prizes and that are rewarded, usually by recognition and status. S/he ambivalently struggles for independence from his/her parents and from all adults. Realistically, however, s/he remains a child, and it is only through identification with his/her peers that s/he is able to feel some of the strength s/he desires. S/he will therefore wish to be an integral part of the peer group. Characteristically, the peer group will exclude those individuals who deviate from its established behavioral and attitudinal norms. The group, in attempting to establish an identity that is unique and independent, tends to seek similarity and conformity among its members. Thus, the emotionally disturbed child whose behavior deviates from the norms of the group will usually be avoided. This contributes to the child's feelings of isolation and prevents him/her from being able to develop rewarding social relations or beginning to achieve independence from his/her home and family.

As the behavior of the emotionally disturbed child becomes more and more inflexible, repetitive, and disruptive and his/her treatment by his/her peers more critical, the school finds itself unable to exert influence by the usual techniques—praise, punishment, affection, or social control. Often this increases the anxieties of the teachers and school administrators in managing the child and induces a feeling of hopelessness on the part of the school. It is usually at this point that the school begins to seek other, more adequate placements for the child. If his/her family living situation is judged to be a major contributing factor to his/her emotional problems and it is felt that his/her progress in another educational setting would be impeded by his/her remaining at home full time, a recommendation for residential or psychiatric hospital inpatient or day care treatment will be made.

When the child becomes an inpatient or day care resident of a psychiatric hospital, his/her formal education continues to be of concern, not only to his/her parents and the public school educators, but the hospital staff as well. For the most part, these people believe that schooling is not an expendable activity of childhood, but rather an activity that is indispensable to normal and healthy adjustment. Therefore, provision is made to continue the child's education while s/he undergoes treatment in the hospital. In some settings, individual tutors are made available to the child. But in growing numbers of psychiatric hospital programs, psychoeducational school programs exist and function as integral components of the total treatment milieu.

When the child arrives at the hospital, s/he finds him/herself in a strange, new world, run in different ways by different sorts of people than s/he has known before. Some continuity remains, however: physicians, nurses, and psychiatric technicians assume the responsibility for parental care and supervision. The hospital school and teacher become the counterpart of the public school teacher. Forness and Langdon (1974) and Hewett (1967) have stated that for all children, particularly those with a previously unsatisfying school experience, a good hospital school becomes an essential part of treatment. It is an experience with great ego-building potentials, since it is oriented to reality and allows the child to engage in reality testing. It aims toward the development of skill mastery with individually designed programs based on each child's interests, needs, learning levels and styles, and cognitive strengths and deficits.

By allowing the child to be successful at whatever level of ability s/he is functioning, it aids in the development of self-image and self-esteem and helps him/her to overcome his/her feelings of failure and frustration associated with past school experiences. It enables him/her to learn to handle limits in a nonthreatening, supportive environment. It offers numerous opportunities for him/her to develop more appropriate modes of expression, both verbal and behavioral, and to achieve greater impulse control. It utilizes, in successive stages of development and improvement in the child, varying amounts of group participation and group identification, depending on his/her strengths and needs at the time. This provides him/her with opportunities to develop more satisfying peer relationships. Since many emotionally disturbed children will eventually leave the hospital and go back to their homes and communities on a full-time basis and attend public school, the hospital school plays a major role in preparing them for a successful return. It also aids those children for whom a new educational placement will be sought and contributes to the selection process.

Edith Clark (1969) has written that if the hospital school is to provide the aforementioned opportunities for the growth and education of emotionally disturbed children, the teacher must be viewed as a central and dynamic member of the interdisciplinary team. Traditionally, the teacher's role has not been portrayed as one of equality or dynamic participation with other members of the treatment team. In many situations the team members interacted with each other, directing their requests to the teachers, who were at the receiving end of this communication system. The teacher then had to take the compendium of thought and translate it into pertinent classroom procedure, with the added task of "thinking on her feet." In some instances the role of the teacher was subtly reduced until many of the planned classroom activities and the procedures were the products and judgments of nonteachers. The inference was that generalizations appropriate for psychologists, psychiatrists, and social workers were also appropriate for or could be adequately communicated to and adopted by teachers. Under these conditions, the teacher could not effectively carry out his/her role, and the school program was limited in terms of its treatment value.

According to Edith Clark (1969) hospital programs today that utilize the school as a therapeutic tool recognize the importance of the clinical functions the teacher performs, the wealth of valuable information s/he can provide to the rest of the clinical team, and view him/her as an equal colleague. In addition, they hold the view that the teacher's role is to enable the child to move toward positive ego growth and to help him/her acquire and experience feelings as an accepted, knowing, and confident self in relation to his/her world.

The author's extensive professional experience enables her to state that the educational therapist must develop the following competencies:

To educate the other members of the interdisciplinary team about his/her role and responsibilities and the objectives of the classroom structure and activities

To understand the theoretical frame of reference of each professional discipline, participating in the team and the language common to each

To be knowledgeable about theories of child development, cognitive and intellectual development, and curriculum development

To utilize a variety of educational diagnostic tools and be familiar with currently published educational materials and equipment

To put into operation principles of group process and techniques for initiating and facilitating group participation

To selectively use different motivational and reinforcement techniques

To evaluate the effectiveness of the programs, strategies, and techniques implemented and make changes when warranted

To be aware of his/her feelings about each student and to relate objectively with individuals of different personality types

To seek consultation or supervision when indicated

The primary tool with which the teacher works is in the individualized educational program designed for each student based on his/her capacities, needs, and efficiency level of ego functioning. The physical environment in which the educational program is implemented has an impact upon its effectiveness. Therefore, the teacher should play an active role in selecting the classroom space, furniture, and interior decorations best suited to the needs of the students. If these factors have been decided upon prior to hiring the teacher, it is important that s/he be able to make whatever changes or additions are necessary.

In the majority of the psychiatric hospital school programs described in the literature and those in which the author has either participated or observed, the planning phase of the educational program for each child is essentially similar. It is conducted by the teacher with input provided by other team members and consists of an initial period of observation and evaluation. This enables an assessment to be made of the child's social/emotional, academic, and cognitive skills and levels of functioning. During this time, the teacher will arrange to meet with the child either on the living unit or in the classroom to review past school history and experiences and to encourage externalization of positive and negative feelings about these experiences. In addition, the student's interests and hobbies are explored and educational testing is conducted. Psychological testing by a licensed psychologist may also occur during this time period. The teacher may observe the child on the living unit to gain further insight about his/her use of language and other communication skills, auditory acuity, primary ways of exploring the world, ability to explore and fruitfully use equipment and objects, skill in using his/her body, and, generally, intellectual functioning and potential. The social worker will formulate a biopsychosocial assessment of the child to include his/her current interrelationships with family members, family views toward the value and importance of education, and sibling school performance. If occupational and recreational therapists are members of the treatment team, they will begin to work with the child in individual and/or group situations.

After the observation period has ended, the team members will meet to share their findings. The teacher will then exercise his/her particular skill in developing an individualized educational plan for the child based on all relevant case material presented. This will include short- and long-term academic and behavioral objectives, proposed curriculum, and educational materials and equipment to be used. The teacher will then meet with the student to review the educational plan. A discussion of the behavioral expectations for the student and school group as a whole is usually included, as well as a visit to the classroom if this has not already occurred. The child will then begin to attend the school program on a full-time basis, unless a modified schedule is necessary to meet his/her individual needs.

During the school day, much time is devoted to individual work periods during which the child learns, through varying amounts of interaction with the teacher, to master the academic and behavioral skills designated in his/her programs. Group activities are also conducted for this purpose as well as to foster whatever peer interaction may be possible. These activities may include group discussions, structured lessons, games, musical activities, art projects, movies, field trips, and recreational activities.

The teacher must often initiate group activities and invite voluntary participation. S/he should choose activities that will not be overstimulating for some of the children but that will maintain an attractive and inviting learning environment, and s/he should always support the children in their efforts to move toward new experiences. By providing carefully selected materials and offering adequate arrangements for their use in the context of a group situation, the classroom provides a fertile ground for the development of more satisfactory and satisfying peer relationships.

While attempting to live within a group of his/her peers, an emotionally disturbed child often demands concentrated attention from an accepting and sympathetic person. The teacher can help the child to discover that s/he can be used in a variety of ways, from providing a temporary symbiotic tie to simply offering momentary support to help the child succeed. S/he can also help the child learn to delay his/her need for immediate attention and gratification and share him/ her with the other students.

Many of the children in the class may not be able to handle limits effectively, as they have not lived in an environment where limits are consistently set. As a result, they may grow desperate at times in their efforts to find protection boundaries. When the classroom is structured in such a way that all rules and expectations are clearly understood and limits consistently set by the teacher, the children are able to feel safe and secure and, in turn, develop more adaptive behavior.

At times, a child may be temporarily unable or unwilling to exert sufficient self-control to meet the expectations of the classroom and will require a "time out" period. The teacher will choose either to spend the time with the student in a designated area away from the classroom or ask the nursing staff to escort the student back to the living unit, where an exploration of the difficulties encountered in the classroom will occur. As soon as the issues are clarified and resolved sufficiently to allow the child to regain control of his/her behavior, s/he will be encouraged to return to the classroom. This process provides additional opportunities for him/her to develop greater ability to verbalize feelings and to gain some insight into his/her behavior and its consequences.

For those children who have previously experienced failure in school, the teacher can help them relive those experiences in a less destructive and more supportive way, identify their feelings about those experiences, and learn to integrate them. By developing individualized reward systems based on each child's level of emotional functioning, the teacher can encourage poorly motivated and/or failure-ridden children to attempt to perform in school. This will enable them to begin to view themselves as learners and to experience the social and emotional gains this role provides.

By continuing to observe and evaluate the behavior of the children in the classroom, the teacher is able to make changes in the group and individual educational programs when necessary. Detailed records of the students' progress will enable him/her to evaluate the effectiveness of the techniques and strategies employed.

As the children spend a major portion of each day in the school program, the interrelationships that form and the psychodynamic and academic issues that arise and are dealt with have an impact on their behavior in other areas of the treatment program. Individual and group issues that occur on the living unit also influence the students' behavior in the classroom. As a result, a well-organized communication system between the teacher and the other members of the treatment team is essential, and it requires the following procedures.

Prior to the beginning of each school day, the teacher receives information about the physical and emotional status of each student from the nursing staff, either in written or verbal form. During the course of the school day, designated nursing staff are available to assist the teacher in dealing with students who require a "time out" period. At the conclusion of the school day, the teacher records information about the daily intellectual and social functioning of each student in the form of progress notes, which are made available to all staff members. In addition, a verbal summary may be given to designated nursing staff to be incorporated in the change of shift report.

The teacher is available to meet with the individual members of a child's treatment team to discuss pertinent issues when necessary. S/he meets with the students' parents upon request to discuss school-related issues. S/he participates in clinical conferences concerning the students and scheduled team meetings.

When a child's discharge date approaches, the teacher has an important role in making a decision regarding an appropriate school placement, taking into account the needs of the child and the available educational resources. Placement may range from a regular classroom in a public school to special classes or even a private residential school. Considerable effort should be expended toward securing appropriate educational placement, since the right match between a child's level of readiness and the class in which s/he is ultimately placed is crucial to his/her subsequent school success. A final report is prepared by the teacher detailing educational and behavioral levels, progress, and behavioral and educational approaches likely to be successful in the school to which the child is being referred. The teacher is available for necessary consultation with the ongoing setting.

In summary, the role of the teacher in a psychiatric hospital school setting is complex and demanding. S/he strives to create and implement individualized educational programs in a climate that fosters motivation, learning, and growth. S/he contributes to the total therapeutic milieu by helping to meet the children's emotional and social needs, including the need for achievement and success, for structure, stable relationships, healthy identification, and appropriate expression of feelings. S/he attempts to arrange an effective school placement following discharge through participation in the selection process and the follow-up program, involving close liaison with the staff members involved in the therapeutic treatment program. For only through such teamwork is it possible to achieve the mutual goals of both the hospital and school; namely, to make it possible for the child to eventually become a more healthy, productive, and participating member of society.

REFERENCES

Cohen, S. How to alleviate first year shock of teaching emotionally disturbed children. *Children*, Vol. 13(6), pp. 232–236, (1966).

Colvin, R.W. The education of emotionally disturbed children in a residential treatment center. Paper presented at the Annual Meeting for Educational Programming for Emotionally Disturbed Children, Syracuse, New York (1960).

Dapper, G. *Educating Children with Special Needs; Current Trends in School Policies and Programs.* National School Public Relations Associations, Arlington, Va. (1974).

Forness, S., and Langdon, F. School in the psychiatric hospital. *Journal of the American Academy of Child Psychiatry, 13*, p. 562–575 (1974).

Grace, H.K. *The Development of a Child Psychiatric Treatment Program.* Schenhman, New York (1974), pp. 25–60.

Halpern, W.I., and Kissel, S. *Human Resources for Troubled Children.* Wiley, New York (1978), pp. 149–174.

Hewett, F. Establishing a school in a psychiatric hospital. *Mental Hygiene, 51*, 275–284 (1967).

Knobloch, P. Toward a broader concept of the role of the special class for emotionally disturbed children. *Exceptional Children, 31*(7), 329–335 (1964).

Love, H.D. *Educating Exceptional Children in a Changing Society.* Charles C Thomas, Springfield (1974), pp. 301–327.

Schultz, E.W., Brown, M.E., and Cohn, R. Educational services in psychiatric and residential programs. *Child Welfare, 52*, 573–584 (1973).

Taylor, E.C. Out of the classroom: Teachers Role In a Therapeutic Pre-School, *Exceptional Children*, Vol. 36(4), 273–276 (Dec. 1969).

Walsh, B. A network of services for severely disturbed adolescents. *Child Welfare, 58*, 115–125 (1979).

10

Recognition and Treatment
of Child Sexual Abuse

Roland Summit

INTRODUCTION

Sexual abuse is the last frontier in the growing awareness of child abuse (Sgroi, 1975). Common knowledge, clinical traditions, and much of the current practice in dealing with child victims of sexual abuse are based on a persistent mythology that serves to minimize effective intervention and potential recovery. The myths are perpetuated by what Sandra Butler (1979) has called "a conspiracy of silence" that insulates adult society against confronting the terrifying discovery that large numbers of children are molested, incestuously assaulted, exploited, and raped by their entrusted caretakers.

No one can welcome such a discovery. The most caring adult and the most dedicated clinician will cling to the mythical hope that incest is rare, that "good" families are immune, and that "normal" men would not sexually exploit children. It is somehow easier to accept that children imagine or exaggerate accounts of sexual abuse, or that the intrinsic sexuality of children makes them irresistibly seductive.

Psychiatrists and other behavioral scientists have been trained to recognize oedipal conflicts and wish-fulfilling behaviors in children. These are accepted as normal and universal. Adult pedophilic behavior, on the other hand, tends to be defined as stereotypic and confined to specifically disturbed characters, with an implicit expectation that such character pathology would be self-revealing and readily diagnosed.

When an apparently normal child presents with implications of sexual involvement with an apparently normal adult the logical conclusions are almost inescapable. Either nothing has happened (the child imaged it) or the normal adult has been victimized by a seductive child.

These conclusions are reinforced by the symptomatic behavior of the child and by the convincing denial of the adult involved. It is not unusual for parents to retaliate against their child in defense of a trusted relative or friend. It is also common for an adult offender to rely on character witnesses, psychiatric examination, and psychological testing to prove his normalcy, while an equivocal clinical evaluation of the distressed child is used to impeach the testimony of the child. Finally, and most unfortunately, it is all too common for the child to equivocate, to deny, or to take the blame for the sexual encounters out of fear of adult retaliation and in the scathing self-judgment and self-punishment typical of the abused child.

Physicians are given an awesome responsibility and an exalted expectation of knowledge and competence in an area where they have very little specific training or experience. Recognition, belief, support, and protective advocacy for the sexually abused child depend on an awareness of new, still-controversial data and a willingness to question a number of cherished, very comforting levels of denial. The basic task is defined by Suzanne Sgroi (1975, p. 20), an internist who is one of the pioneering physicians in the field of child abuse:

> Recognition of sexual molestation of a child is entirely dependent on the individual's inherent willingness to entertain the possibility that the condition may exist. Unfortunately, willingness to consider the diagnosis of suspected child sexual molestation frequently seems to vary in inverse proportion to the individual's level of training. That is, the more advanced the training of some, the less willing they are to suspect molestation.

The physician who is prepared to believe in the realities of child sexual abuse takes on the task of dealing with resistance at a personal, intrapsychic level as well as to the intraprofessional and interprofessional levels. Dr. Sgroi (1978, p. xv) speaks from long and painful experience:

> Those who try to assist sexually abused children must be prepared to battle against incredulity, hostility, innuendo, and outright harassment. Worst of all, the advocate for the sexually abused child runs the risk of being smothered by indifference and a conspiracy of silence. The pressure from one's peer group as well as the community, to ignore, minimize, or cover up the situation may be extreme.

The physician has the opportunity for uniquely definitive intervention on behalf of mental health. Sexual abuse has been called a "psychological time bomb" (Peters, 1973), which can be totally destructive to later adult adjustment even when the child has shown no immediate signs of emotional trauma. Self-hate; self-destructive, antisocial behaviors; substance abuse; running away; prostitution; somatic complaints; sexual dysfunctions; hysterical seizures; dissociative disorders, including multiple personality states and homicidal frenzies; affective disorders; and schizophrenia—all may be associated with sexual abuse.

While it is obvious that sexual abuse itself is not the sole cause of every kind of identity crisis or emotional disorder and that not all victims of sexual abuse are equally disabled, recent clinical experience inspires some radical claims. There is no question that specific therapeutic resolution of incest trauma can provide dramatic remissions of major mental illness and behavior disorders in appropriately selected cases. The possibility of a single-trauma etiology in these patients raises promise for primary prevention of mental illness if sexual abuse crises can be resolved during childhood.

As in other forms of child abuse, there is a generational bonus of prevention if a victim can be identified and reparented. In a substantial proportion of cases, today's victim is tomorrow's offender. Boy victims tend to grow up to molest other boys. Girls can become part of an "incest carrier syndrome" (Berry, 1977), unable to protect their daughters from the incest-prone men they seem compelled to select. Uncounted numbers of children in future generations can be spared the geometric chain reaction of abuse for each link that can be broken through effective intervention and care.

Child sexual abuse therefore presents to the physician as a confusing and threatening enigma that invites denial, avoidance, and rejection. For the clinician with the foresight and courage to confront the problems of sexual abuse and to become a part of the solution, the therapeutic and preventive rewards can be profound.

SCOPE OF SEXUAL ABUSE

Sexual abuse is anything but exotic or rare. It is an everyday sort of experience for hundreds of thousands of children in every economic and cultural subgroup in the United States. While other forms of child abuse are limited to immediate caretakers, sexual abuse may be initiated by parents, live-in partners, extended-family members, friends, community caretakers, even strangers.

Retrospective surveys indicate that at least 20–30 percent of females experience some sort of sexual victimization before age 13 (Landis, 1956; Gagnon, 1965; Finkelhor, 1979a). These and other studies (Weiss et al., 1955; DeFrancis, 1969; Benward and Densen-Gerber, 1975; Peters, 1976; Queen's Bench, 1976; Burgess et al., 1978) are consistent in a startling observation: only 25 percent of the offenders are strangers. A girl who has been taught to beware of strangers is totally unprepared for the three-to-one chance that she will be approached by someone she has been taught to trust and obey. Forty-four percent of all victim experiences were with family members, including 22 percent within the child's household. Six percent of all victimizing relationships were with fathers or stepfathers (Finkelhor, 1979a). The figures in Finkelhor's survey of college students are predictably conservative. Projecting that sample to the general population suggests that at least nine percent of all women were sexually victimized by an older relative, with some two percent involved in sex with their fathers or step-fathers.

Numbers for males are more elusive. Boys are known to be even more reluctant than girls to admit to sexual victimization. In Finkelhor's survey (1979*a*) half as many males as females reported childhood sexual victimization. Only 25 percent of the boys told anyone during the time victimization occurred, compared to 38 percent of the girls in the same sample. There is good reason to believe that boys are even more frequently engaged in sex with adults than are girls, since they are the preferred target of habitual pedophiles (Groth, 1978). No survey is any better than the ability of the victims to define and to confide their experiences. After a concerted effort to educate Detroit school children to report sexual molestation, the ratio of boys to girls reporting rose from a baseline of 1:6 to 1:1 (Groth, 1980).

Any community or clinical response system that acts to end the secrecy and denial surrounding sexual abuse will be confronted with an explosive increase in the apparent incidence. Santa Clara County in California, which initiated the model Child Sexual Abuse Treatment Project, has experienced a 30,000 percent increase in the reporting of sexual abuse over the past seven years (Giaretto, 1980)!

Peeling away layers of secrecy uncovers not only unexpected numbers, but also increasingly disturbing realities of the victimization process. We can no longer reassure ourselves that victims are consenting or seductive partners who share responsibility with adults. Latency-age children, not nubile adolescents, are the most frequent victims. The average girl victim is eight at the time of initiation, and many are only two or three years old. In one nonclinical sample of 183 women who had experienced incest, 180 were *under eight* when the sexual activity began (Armstrong, 1978). The so-called seductive years are almost immune: girls over 13 rarely allow incestuous relationships. Boys are most at risk in the three or four years immediately preceding puberty, roughly 9–13. These are naive children who are intimidated by the intrinsic power of an adult. The adult offers acceptance, affection, and security on the one hand and threatens rejection, punishment, and chaos on the other. While overt violence and physical injury are the exceptions, intimidation, coercion, and threats are basic to the sexual misuse of children by adults.

Nor are the sexual experiences themselves the stuff of romantic or seductive dreams. The words "fondle" or "caress" are often used to describe moves better characterized as grab, rub, probe, lick, and suck. Whenever children are given permission to break the silence and to offer explicit descriptions, they talk of beings used as accessories to sexual demands of adults, with almost no hint of gentleness, playfulness, titillation, reciprocity, affection, or even explanations or reassurances (Burgess and Holmstrom, 1975). The eight-year-old girl who describes being awakened at night to take her father's penis in her mouth, gagging on the semen and being forced to swallow it, is hardly conjuring up an oedipal fantasy.

Since the girl is sexually undeveloped and since the man generally tries to avoid physical injury, vaginal intercourse is usually not the immediate goal. Manual, oral, or anal containment of the penis are the "normal" activities of incestuous intercourse, as they are also for the more typically out-of-family sexual misuse of boys.

Although both girls and boys may be the targets of sexual abuse, the adult is almost invariably male. While women are at least equally capable of other forms of child abuse, including physical battery, neglect, and verbal and emotional abuse, they seem better able than men to respect the sexual autonomy of children in their care. This should not be too surprising, since it merely reinforces a truism in sexual perversity: compulsive voyeurs, exhibitionists, fetishists, pedophiles, rapists, sex murderers, and other mentally disordered sex offenders are males. Occasional exceptions occur, of course, and these atypical women become celebrated and immortalized in popular literature. They are the exotic exceptions that prove the rule. Sexually perverse males are not newsworthy. We seem to take it for granted that men will almost normally sexualize their need for power or subordinate others to their need for sex, no matter how eccentric or odious that need might be. Robert Stoller (1974), one of the premier psychoanalysts in the field of gender identity and sexual behavior, believes that perverse mechanisms are almost inevitable in the development of male sexuality.

DEFINITIONS

Sexual abuse is not necessarily incest, nor is incest necessarily abusive. Incest is a legal term defining sexual intercourse between two persons so closely related that they are forbidden by law to marry. In that narrow sense, coitus between first cousins at age 20 is incest, while oral copulation between a four-year-old and her father is not. Incest between siblings seems to be harmless in many cases if the relationship is free from intimidation and if there is no punitive discovery by adults. As a clinical issue, then, we are concerned not with consanguinity as much as with age-power relationships and the betrayal of a trusted, caretaking role. We are also concerned less with technicalities of penetration or genital touching than with the child's sense that he or she has been sexually violated.

Sexual abuse in the context of the present discussion is defined as the involvement of a child in specifically sexual activities with an adult. While I believe that such involvement is likely to be harmful, it is not necessary to demonstrate immediate damage in the child or even to prove that all intergenerational sexual contact is ultimately harmful. It should be enough to understand unequivocally that sexualization of a child-caring relationship is, in itself, a violation of ethics. As David Finkelhor (1979*b*) argues so simply and yet so eloquently, a child is incapable of informed consent with a controlling adult. The child has no power to say no and has no information on which to base a decision. Since the long-term effects are so uncertain, and since the adult has such a vested interest in minimizing those risks, no modern concept of ethics, liability, or consumer protection could ever endorse such a lopsided contract. The child is just as powerless within the intimidating or ingratiating relationship as the adult rape victim would be at the point of a knife.

PATTERNS OF SEXUAL ABUSE

Motivation for sexual abuse of children ranges from trivial impulses to ritualistic compulsions (Summit and Kryso, 1978). No single clinical paradigm can be defined. Most offenders are relatively indifferent to the needs and feelings of children, even though the adult may see himself as uniquely caring and devoted to his child love. Many of the categories in the clinical spectrum differ from one another largely in the degree of power, punishment, and perversity imposed on the child. These variations in parental motivation and behavior are discussed more thoroughly in "Sexual Abuse of Children: A Clinical Spectrum" (Summit and Kryso, 1978). The most important distinction for treatment planning and estimation of prognosis is the differential diagnosis between pedophilia and endogamous incest.

Nicholas Groth (1978) defines a very practical and consistent dichotomy between *fixated* and *regressed* offenders.

The Fixated Offender

The fixated offender remains fixed at a preadolescent level of sexual object choice.* He fails to find comfort or confidence in sexual relationships with age-mates beyond puberty. Immature partners provide a continuing attraction which typically comes to resemble a compulsion or addiction. In addition to the compelling erotic appeal, the fixated offender sees children as preferred objects of

---

*Such a fixation can result from trauma, as in a preadolescent sexual assault, or from excessive stimulation, such as an affectionate childhood relationship with a pedophile. In other cases there is no discernible basis for the fixation. As with other types of sexual paraphilias, theories of etiology remain diverse and controversial. Whatever the causes may be, it is important to recognize that pedophilia can exist as a disorder of sexual object coice without associated disorders of thought, affect, or behavior.

companionship and love. Most such men are kind and indulgent in the extreme with their partners, never resorting to physical force or injury. They may spend years developing an affectionate, trusted relationship with the child and the parents. Children and their adult caretakers are disarmed by the uncommon interest and empathy offered by these men, who may also gain occupational positions of unquestioned trust and authority with children. A fixated offender may function very effectively as a physician, police officer, minister, youth worker, teacher, coach, or "good neighbor Sam." While offenders studied in prison populations tend to be ineffectual and poorly socialized, there are large numbers of lifetime pedophiles who are never reported, convicted, nor even suspected by friends and neighbors. They may be married (preference for children does not rule out a capacity for genital performance with adults), highly respected, well employed, and completely reliable and ethical to all outward appearances.

The fixated offender has a lifetime to accommodate to this affiliation with children, and he may escape any feelings of guilt or remorse. He tends to develop an eccentric rationalization that children desire and need his love and that he has a mission to rescue them from the distant, uncaring world of ordinary adults. His child partners often reinforce that view, since he seeks children who are starved for attention and affection (Martin, 1980). Such needy children may accommodate with active curiosity and without complaint to the sexual games introduced by their special friend.

While the rationalization of guiltlessness may be defined as sociopathic, it can also be seen as analogous to the eccentric mores that are vital for the survival of any persecuted minority group. For instance, political terrorism, assassination, execution, war, and euthanasia can extend permission to otherwise ethical individuals to kill one another. The fixated offender presents an impossible dilemma to any rigid diagnostic scheme. Any clinician who insists that an offender against children must be sociopathic, psychotic, antisocial, or sadistic will simply refuse to recognize the well-adjusted, beguiling, professional molester of children. The "well-adjusted" pedophile can elude any clinical measure of psychopathology. Clinical interviews, mental status testing, standardized testing, projective testing, even polygraph examination will give no hint of emotional discomfort or psychopathology.

The fixated offender, or habitual pedophile, tends to be fixed to the sexual object most characteristic of preadolescence: his male playmates. The vast majority of habitual pedophiles are attracted exclusively to boys. A small minority seeks girls exclusively. Ambisexual pedophilia is relatively rare. This predominant attraction to boys should not be confused with homosexuality. When the so-called boy lover has any sexual interest in an adult, the age-mate will be a woman. None of the men in Groth's (1978) sample had any adult homosexual experience.

Those fixated offenders who prefer young females have restricted opportunity for unchallenged association with girls. Since an unrelated male is less likely to be trusted as a coach or other group caretaker of girls, the typical mode of operation for the female-specific pedophile is to seek out lonely, vulnerable mothers who are looking for a father figure for their daughters. Finkelhor (1979c) found that girls who had stepfathers were five times more likely than average to be sexually victimized. In fact, fully 50 percent of the stepdaughters in the sample acknowledge childhood victimization. The sexual contact was most often not with the stepfather himself but with more transient predators who capitalized on the vulnerability of a broken family. Like the well-adjusted boy lover, the habitual molester of girls tends to be highly gifted in inspiring trust and gratitude in beleaguered mothers. It is not uncommon for mothers to send their daughters on day-long and even overnight excursions with a prospective stepfather, as if to test and insure their compatability.

The fixated offender tends to have a rather narrowly circumscribed age-preference range. He knows that his love affair with a given child is time limited and that his compelling sexual attraction will turn to indifference or even repulsion within a few years. The appearance in the child of secondary sexual characteristics is like the stroke of midnight for Cinderella. The experienced pedophile learns to replace the fading attraction of each relationship with a succession of younger initiates. An active pedophile may have contact with hundreds, even thousands of children within his lifetime (Martin, 1980)!

The Regressed Offender

The regressed offender is the typical incest offender. The individual has followed a normal progression of adjustments to age-mate sexual partners. He was not aware of selective fantasy or sexual attraction related to children. Neither does he have any particular interest in or empathy with the world of children. When habitual and preferred adult relationships become conflicted and if he feels threatened and ineffectual in his adult adjustment, he is likely to seek endorsement and a sense of importance through the sexualization of a relationship with a more available, more subordinate, and less threatening partner. The man rather suddenly and unexpectedly finds his child irresistible for a variety of reasons: (1) the child is available in a preexisting, totally subordinate, intimate reationship; (2) the child is affectionate, trusting, and attentive—eager to gain more acceptance, endorsement, and affectionate expression from the father; (3) the child embodies many of the mannerisms and appearances typical of the mother at an earlier, more idealized stage of the marriage—a kind of reincarnation of the breathless, responsive, adoring partner in adolescent courtship relationships; (4) the child, as a part of the mother, is an attractive foil for punishment and revenge in the frustration of the marital relationship; and (5) the potential for sexuality in the child is seen by the father as a threat to innocence and the beginnings of degradation and/or rebellious alientation from parental control. This fear of eventual autonomy for the child and the dread of out-of-family seduction seems to prompt extreme possessiveness and a compulsion for extraordinary measures of control, including perverse examples of hands-on "sex education."

These factors, and many other more idiosyncratic variables, are most selective for the female child as a surrogate for and a target of regression from the previous adjustment with a female age-mate. The regressed offender will be involved less often with boys and least often with both girls and boys (Groth, 1978).

The initial regressive experience or attraction is often experienced as overwhelming—beyond the conscious wish or control of the offender. The attraction does not make sense to him, and his conscious defenses are dominated by denial, projection, and dissociation. He may also be depressed, desperate, and relatively uncaring. His need for assurance of his own adequacy reassures him there is no crisis he can't control; so he avoids confiding in anyone for help. He tends to believe he is responding appropriately to the seduction or provocation of a willing partner.

Dissociative aspects are quite variable, allowing for a suspension of prevailing roles. The man in the process of regression acts as if he were young and powerful again, smitten with an excitingly youthful partner. He sees the child as old enough and in need of sexual attention, no matter what her actual age or level of development. He may see her as the direct embodiment of her mother or some other lost love object. Or he may conceptualize his sexual coercion as not at all sexual, but rather as necessary parental exercises in education or discipline. There is a fine line here between regression, dissociation, distortion, delusion, rationalization, and plain, old-fashioned self-justification. Whatever the relative mix of psychodynamic and psychopathological variables, most regressed offenders do not test out clinically as psychotic, borderline, hysterical, sociopathic, or sexually deviant. In terms of measurable psychopathology, the regressed offender is technically normal.

After a sexual encounter the offender may be filled with guilt, remorse, fear, and anger and he will tend to blame the child for his distress. Because of the inherent conflicts and the essentially ego-alien nature of the attraction, the regressed offender has little capacity to invite friendly, leisurely, potentially gratifying peer-level relationships with the child. He forces the child into adult styles of behavior and holds her to adult levels of accountability and responsibility. Control and submissiveness are inherent in the preexisting parent-child relationship; so he insures silence more often by intimidation and threat than by ingratiation.

Once the taboo against incest and adult-child sexuality has been broken, and once the offender is plagued with a recurring cycle of need, arousal, gratification, and punishment, the behavior may become habitual and compulsive. While the regressed offender is unlikely to premeditate and create new sexual relationships with unrelated children, any children within his sphere of authority may be at risk once a pattern is established. The regressed offender who serially involves his younger children and eventually even his grandchildren will rarely attempt contacts outside of the family.

Some regressed offenders find their initiation outside of a parental controlling relationship, being attracted to a child who is a close family friend or a devoted student. Therefore not every teacher, minister, or coach who molests a child is a fixated or habitual offender. Conversely, not every predation within a family represents a regressive response to a crisis in adult adjustment. Seduction of a family member may be part of a long-term pedophilic compulsion. There is no blood barrier to pedophilic intrusion. Differential diagnosis depends on an accurate assessment of the lifetime adjustment patterns of the offender.

The clinical assessment of anyone accused of sexual activity with a child *must* draw on every possible source of collateral data, including marital, employment, and arrest records. *The history presented by the offender has no bearing on any behavior that he may choose to conceal.* While this fact should be obvious, it is ignored again and again in clinical evaluations that rule out pedophilia and that declare that a man is normal because he says he has never been attracted to children.

Accurate assessment of the offender is of more than academic interest. Prognosis for treatment and control of pedophilic behavior is diametrically opposed in the two groups. Despite the hopes of penologists and therapists, there is no responsible documentation that treatment can realign the sexual preference of the fixated pedophile or gain any protection for the children at risk. Since the well-adjusted pedophile typically finds an unrestricted supply of noncomplaining partners, there is no means short of 24-hour supervision to monitor the effectiveness of any outpatient treatment model.

Finally, the lifetime pattern of ego-syntonic adjustment, missionary enthusiasm, and pressure for survival give intense energy to an illicit pedophile subculture. The pedophile underworld has its own literature, communication network, economic vested interests (child pornography and prostitution), and elitist philosophies. The pedophile subculture serves not only to reinforce the safety and comfort of pedophiles but to minimize public concern for the protective needs of children and for the need for more effective control and treatment of pedophilia. Naturally, the overt and covert political efforts of such organizations as the North American Man-Boy Love Association (NAMBLA) rally in support of the most ineffectual, least repressive control and treatment programs, while graduates of the treatment programs are profuse in their praise and gratitude for their "recovery." In summary, there is little theoretical hope for treatment and no objective measure of treatment outcome for the fixated offender.

In contrast, the regressed offender has an excellent prognosis and a vital need for the specialized treatment that can provide total recovery. Treatment results can be monitored through follow-up within the predictable scope of potential victims. Rehabilitation is facilitated by reinforcement of preexisting family resources and appropriate adult sexual relationships, especially since the typical regressed offender is so intensely motivated to recover those resources and relationships. Since a familial bond defines most of those relationships, the treatment program has access to all parties to the sexual disturbance, with the opportunity for parallel treatment, peer-group reinforcement, and resocialization of the individuals as well as the family units. Since there is little subcultural organization or support for incest, and since accommodation to child sexual objects has been more recent and more ego-dystonic for the offender, conventional ethics and societal mores can be drawn upon to reinforce child-protective and adult-developmental values within therapeutic groups. Even if there were only minimal growth and recovery in the offender, child victims and their mothers could be so strengthened through treatment that they would no longer tolerate sexual exploitation. Therapy for the regressed offender is both theoretically justified and empirically demonstrated. Most important, therapy can be objectively monitored and extended in preventive continuity to potential victims.

It should not be assumed that offenders of either type will present themselves willingly or openly for diagnosis, nor that they will invest themselves in voluntary treatment. The regressed offender will mobilize every available dodge and alibi to evade personal, professional, or public recognition of his problem. The potential for recovery can be realized only within the context of absolute prohibition of any sexual access to children, with enough coercive leverage to overpower any hope of hiding or of continuing regressive and exploitive sexual relationships. The structures and techniques of this delicate balance of coercion and support will be further explored in the section on treatment.

ROLE OF THE CHILD

The normal behavior of a child caught up in sexual abuse creates alienation and prejudice in potential caregivers. These normal adjustment patterns must be understood before the clinician can be an effective advocate for abused children. The full syndrome of accommodation is most characteristic of incestuous abuse; so a father-daughter paradigm will be described. Many of the same reactions can be seen in ongoing out-of-family molestations as well. The child sexual abuse accommodation syndrome includes five characteristics: secrecy, helplessness, accommodation, delayed disclosure, and retraction.

Secrecy

Children rarely tell anyone, especially when they are first molested (Finkel-hor, 1979a; Burgess and Holmstrom, 1975). The child typically feels ashamed and guilty. She fears disapproval or punishment from the mother (most of the girls in Finkelhor's sample who told their mothers found their worst fears were justified), retaliation or loss of love from the offender, and, most profoundly, loss of acceptance and security in the home. *These fears are often suggested and reinforced by direct threats from the offender.*

The emphasis on secrecy and the fearful isolation from the mother define the sexual activity as something dangerous and bad, even if the child is too young to understand the societal taboos involved. Even if the child is carefully and affectionately seduced without fear or pain, the conspiracy of silence stigmatizes the relationship.

Helplessness

The child feels obligated and overpowered by the inherent authority of the trusted adult, even in the absence of physical force or threats. Helplessness is reinforced by the sense of isolation, secrecy, and guilt, as well as the child's inability to make sense out of her father's behavior or to find any acceptable way to describe the bizarre relationship to others.

Helplessness is often expressed by immobility. If a young girl is molested during sleep, she will typically "play possum." She will not resist nor cry out, even though her mother may be in the next room. A sibling in the same bed may also feign sleep, afraid to become involved.

The natural inability to cry out or to protect herself provides the core of mis-understanding between the victim and the community of adults, as well as the nidus for the child's later self-reprisals. Almost no adult seems willing to believe that a legitimate victim would remain still. She is expected to react with kicks and screams. Attorneys for the offender easily humiliate and confuse the child victim-witness and prejudice the jury with demands for a "normal" protest. Expert testimony on these points is crucial both to vindicate the credibility of the child and to help prevent continuing self-condemnation.

With repeated intrusions the victimized child may lie awake in fright long into the night. Yet if approached, she will remain motionless in a pathetic attempt to protect herself, much as she has learned to hide beneath the covers from imaginary monsters.

Violation of a person's most secure retreat overwhelms ordinary defenses and leads to disillusionment, severe insecurity, and a process of victimization. Well-adjusted adults report lingering terrors and loss of basic well-being after a rape or even a robbery within their bedrooms. Children, who have few defenses at best, are even more vulnerable than adults to the invasion of their beds.

Finally, it must be remembered that the normal child has no real power or voice apart from the enfranchisement given by her parents. These are not older children nor adolescents with strong institutional or peer-group support. How can a third-grader feel anything but helplessness in confronting a sexually insistent father or stepfather? And how can such a small child blame herself for inviting his attentions or for her failure to forcibly abort his intentions? For a child of eight (or three or five or eleven, as the case may be) self-blame is intrinsic to the accommodation process, unless her mother or some alternate caretaker can give her the power to stop the sexual entrapment.

Entrapment and Accommodation

The process of helpless victimization leads the child to exaggerate her own responsibility and eventually to despise herself for her weakness. The child is confronted with two apparent realities: either *she* is bad, deserving of punishment and not worth caring for, or her *parent* is bad, unfairly punishing and not capable of caring. The young child has neither preparation nor permission to believe in the second reality, and there would be no hope for acceptance or survival if it were true. Her inevitable choice is to embrace the more active role of being the one responsible and to hope to find a way to become good and worthy of caring. This self-scapegoating is almost universal for victims of any form of parental abuse. It sets the foundation for self-hate and what Leonard Shengold (1979, p. 539) describes as a vertical split in reality testing:

> If the very parent who abuses and is experienced as *bad* must be turned to for relief of the distress that the parent has caused, then the child must, out of desperate need, register the parent—*delusionally*—as good. Only the mental image of a good parent can help the child deal with the terrifying intensity of fear and rage which is the effect of the tormenting experiences. The alternative—the maintenance of the overwhelming stimulation and the bad parental image—means annihilation of identity, of the feeling of the self. So the bad has to be registered as good. This is a mind-splitting or mind-fragmenting operation.

The sexually abusing parent provides graphic example and instruction in how to be good: the child must be available without complaint to his sexual demands. There is an explicit or implicit promise of reward: if she is good and if she keeps the secret, she can protect her siblings from sexual involvement ("It's a good thing I can count on you to love me; otherwise I'd have to turn to your little sister"), protect her mother from disintegration ("If your mother ever found out, it would kill her"), protect her father from temptation ("If I couldn't count on you, I'd have to hang out in bars and look for other women"), and, most vitally, preserve the security of the home ("If you ever tell, they could send me to jail and put all you kids in an orphanage").

In the classical role reversal of child abuse, the child is given the power to destroy the family and the responsibility to keep it together. The child, *not the parent*, must mobilize the altruism and self-control to insure the survival of the others. The child, in short, must secretly assume many of the role-functions ordinarily assigned to the mother.

There is an inevitable splitting of conventional moral values: maintaining a lie to keep the secret is the ultimate virtue, while telling the truth would be the greatest sin. A child thus victimized will appear to accept or to seek sexual contact without complaint. As Ferenczi discovered almost 50 years ago, "The misused child changes into a mechanical obedient automaton" (1933, p. 163).

Effective accommodation, of course, invalidates any future claims to credibility as a victim. It is obvious to adults that if the child were sexually involved, as she claims, then she must have been a consenting and probably a seductive partner. Otherwise, she would have told right away. Either she is lying in her eventual complaints or she lied and conspired with her "lover" in her earlier cover-up. In either event, she has no credibility in a criminal court. Again, only expert testimony can translate the child's behavior into concepts that other adults can accept.

Since the child must structure her reality to protect the parent, she also finds the means to build pockets of survival where some hope of goodness can find sanctuary. She may turn to imaginary companions for reassurance. She may develop multiple personalities, assigning helplessness and suffering to one, badness and rage to another, sexual power to another, love and compassion to another, and so forth. She may discover altered states of consciousness to shut off pain or to dissociate from her body, as if looking on from a distance at the child suffering the abuse. The same mechanisms that allow psychic survival for the child become handicaps to effective psychological integration as an adult. Victims at any stage of their accommodation deserve sympathetic professional understanding and assurance that their reactions are understandable, psycho-physiological, and reversible, rather than indications of poor reality testing and continuing psychopathology (Reagor, 1980).

If the child cannot create a psychic economy to reconcile the continuing outrage, the intolerance of helplessness and the increasing feelings of rage will seek active expression. For the girl this is most often self-destructive and reinforcing of self-hate: self-mutilation, suicidal behavior, promiscuous sexual activity, and repeated runaways are typical. She may learn to exploit the father for privileges, favors, and material rewards, reinforcing her self-punishing image as whore in the process. She may fight with both parents, but her greatest rage is likely to focus on her mother, whom she blames for driving the father into her bed. She assumes that her mother must know of the sexual abuse and is either too uncaring or too ineffectual to intervene. The failure of the mother-daughter bond reinforces the young woman's distrust of herself as a female and makes her all the more dependent on the pathetic hope of gaining acceptance and protection with an abusive male.

The male victim of sexual abuse is more likely to turn his rage outward in aggressive and antisocial behavior. He is even more intolerant of his helplessness than the female victim, and more likely to rationalize that he is exploiting the relationship for his own benefit. He may cling so tenaciously to an idealized relationship with the adult that he remains fixed at a preadolescent level of sexual object choice, as if trying to keep love alive with an unending succession of young boys. Various admixtures of depression, counterphobic violence, mysogyny (again, the mother is seen as noncaring and unprotective), and rape seem to be part of the legacy of rage endowed in the sexually abused boy.

Substance abuse is an inviting avenue of escape for the victim of either gender. As Barbara Myers (1981) recalls: "On drugs, I could be anything I wanted to be. I could make up my own reality: I could be pretty, have a good family, a nice father, a strong mother, and be happy. . . . Drinking had the opposite effect of drugs. . . . Drinking got me back into my pain; it allowed me to experience my hurt and my anger."

All these accommodation mechanisms—domestic martyrdom, splitting of reality, altered consciousness, hysterical phenomena, delinquency, sociopathy, projection of rage, even self-mutilation—are part of the survival skills of the child. They can be abandoned only if the child can be led to trust in a secure environment that is full of consistent, *noncontingent* acceptance and caring. In the meantime, anyone working therapeutically with the child (or the grown-up, still shattered victim) will be tested and provoked to prove that trust is impossible, and that the only secure reality is negative expectations and self-hate. It is all too easy for the would-be therapist to join the parents and all of adult society in rejecting such a child, looking at the results of abuse to assume that such an impossible wretch must have asked for and deserved whatever punishment has occurred, if indeed the whole problem is not a hysterical or vengeful fantasy.

Delayed, Conflicted, and Unconvincing Disclosure

Most ongoing sexual abuse is *never* disclosed, at least not outside the immediate family (Gagnon, 1965; Finkelhor, 1979a). Treated, reported, or investigated cases are the exception, not the norm. Disclosure is an outgrowth either of overwhelming family conflict, incidental discovery by a third party, or sensitive outreach and community education by child protective agencies.

If family conflict triggers disclosure, it is usually only after some years of continuing sexual abuse and an eventual breakdown of accommodation mechanisms. The victim of incest remains silent until she enters adolescence, when she becomes capable of demanding a more separate life for herself and challenging the authority of her parents. Adolescence also makes the father more jealous and controlling, trying to sequester his daughter against the "dangers" of outside peer involvement. The corrosive effects of accommodation seem to justify any extreme of punishment. What parent would not impose severe restrictions to control running away, drug abuse, promiscuity, rebellion, and delinquency?

After some especially punishing family fight and a belittling showdown of authority by the father, the girl is finally driven by anger to let go of the secret. *She seeks understanding and intervention at the very time she is least likely to find them.* Authorities are put off by the pattern of delinquency and rebellious anger expressed by the girl. Most adults confronted with such a history tend to identify with the problems of the parents in trying to cope with a rebellious teenager. They observe that the girl seems more angry about the immediate punishment than about the sexual atrocities she is alleging. They assume there is no truth to such a fantastic complaint, especially since the girl did not complain years ago when she claims she was forcibly molested. They assume she has invented the story in retaliation against the father's attempts to achieve reasonable control and discipline. The more unreasonable and abusive the triggering punishment, the more they assume the girl would do anything to get away, even to the point of falsely incriminating her father.

Unless specifically trained and sensitized, the average adult, including mothers, relatives, teachers, counselors, doctors, psychotherapists, investigators, prosecutors, defense attorneys, judges, and jurors cannot believe that a normal, truthful child would tolerate incest without immediately reporting, or that an apparently normal father could be capable of repeated, unchallenged sexual molestation of his own daughter. The child of any age faces an unbelieving audience when she complains of ongoing incest. The troubled, angry adolescent risks not only disbelief, but scapegoating, humiliation, and punishment as well.

Not all complaining adolescents appear angry and unreliable. An alternative accommodation pattern exists in which the child succeeds in hiding any indications of conflict. Such a child may be unusually achieving and popular, eager to please both teachers and peers. When the honor student or the captain of the football team tries to describe a history of ongoing sexual involvement with an adult, the adult reaction is all the more incredulous. How could such a thing have happened to such a fine young person? No one so talented and well-adjusted could have been involved in something so sordid. Obviously, it didn't happen or, if it did, it certainly didn't harm the child. So there is no real cause for complaint. Whether the child is delinquent, hypersexual, countersexual, suicidal, hysterical, psychotic, or perfectly well adjusted, and whether the child is angry, evasive, or serene, the immediate affect and the adjustment pattern of the child will be interpreted by adults to invalidate the child's complaint.

The target of boy love is especially misunderstood. He is likely to be regarded as "queer" or sick. Adolescence has forced a crisis of rejection: the boy has outgrown the age preference of the pedophile. Sometimes the boy is hurt and angry enough to speak out, but more often he will try to cope with his betrayal silently and alone. If he does complain, it is not unusual for parents and others to reject the complaint in defense of the trusted neighbor or colleague.

Contrary to popular myth, most mothers are not aware of ongoing sexual abuse. Pedophilic relatives and friends have a way of inspiring trust and gratitude while they offer love and care for the child. Marriage demands considerable blind trust and denial for survival. A woman does not commit her life and security to a man she believes capable of molesting his own children. That basic denial becomes more exaggerated the more the woman herself has been victimized and the more she might feel helpless and worthless in the absense of a protective, accepting male. The "obvious" clues to sexual abuse are usually obvious only in retrospect. Our assumption that the mother "must have known" merely parallels the demand of the child that the mother must be in touch intuitively with invisible and even deliberately concealed family discomfort.

So the mother typically reacts to allegations of sexual abuse with disbelief and protective denial. How could she not have known? How could the child wait so long to tell her? What kind of mother could allow such a thing to happen? What would the neighbors think? As someone substantially dependent on the approval and generosity of the father, the mother in the incestuous triangle is confronted with a mind-splitting dilemma analogous to that of the abused child: either the child is bad and deserving of punishment or the father is bad and unfairly punitive. One of them is lying and unworthy of trust. The mother's whole security and life adjustment and much of her sense of adult self-worth demand a trust in the reliability of her partner. To accept the alternative means annihilation of the family and a large piece of her own identity. Her fear and ambivalence are reassured by the father's logical challenge: "Are you going to believe that lying little slut? Can you believe I would do such a thing? How could something like that go on right under your nose for years? You know we can't trust her out of our sight anymore. Just when we try to clamp down and I get a little tough with her, she comes back with a cock-and-bull story like this. That's what I get for trying to keep her out of trouble!"

Among the small proportion of incest secrets that are shared, most are never divulged outside of the family. Now that professionals are required to report any suspicion of child abuse, increasing numbers of complaints are investigated by protective agencies. Police investigators and protective service workers are now more likely to give credence to the complaint, in which case all the children may be removed immediately into protective custody pending hearing of a dependency petition. In the continuing paradox of a divided judicial system, the juvenile court judge is likely to sustain out-of-home placement in the "preponderance of the evidence" that the child is in danger, while the adult court takes no action on the father's criminal responsibility. Attorneys know that the uncorroborated testimony of a child will not convict a respectable adult. The test in criminal court requires specific proof "beyond reasonable doubt," and every reasonable adult juror will have reason to doubt the child's fantastic claims. Prosecutors are reluctant to subject the child to humiliating cross-examination, just as they are loath to prosecute cases they cannot win; so they typically reject the complaint on the basis of insufficient evidence. *Defense counsel can assure a father that he will not be charged as long as he denies any impropriety and as long as he stays out of treatment.*

Out-of-family pedophiles are also effectively immune from incrimination if they have any amount of prestige. Even if several children have complained, their testimony will be impeached by trivial discrepancies in their accounts or by the countercharge that the children were willing and seductive conspirators.

The absence of criminal charges is tantamount to a conviction of perjury against the victim. "A man is innocent until proven guilty," say adult-protective relatives. "The kid claimed to be molested but there was nothing to it. The police investigated and they didn't even file charges."

As outrageous as it might seem, there is an open season on children for the sexual predator. Unless children can be encouraged to seek immediate intervention and unless there is expert advocacy for the child in the criminal court, the child is abandoned as the helpless custodian of a self-incriminating secret that no responsible adult can believe.

The physician has a crucial role in both early detection and expert courtroom advocacy. The physician must help mobilize skeptical caretakers into a position of belief, acceptance, support, and protection of the child. The physician must first be capable of assuming that same position. The physician who learns to accept the secrecy, the helplessness, the accommodation, and the delayed disclosure may still be alienated by the fifth level of the accommodation syndrome.

Retraction of Complaint

Whatever a child says about incest, she is likely to reverse it. As a young child, she may deny incest when questioned, yet later she may make criminal complaints when moved by anger. Beneath the anger remains the ambivalence of guilt and the martyred obligation to preserve the family. In the chaotic aftermath of disclosure, the child discovers that the bedrock fears and threats underlying the secrecy are true. Her father abandons her and calls her a liar. Her mother doesn't believe her or she decompensates into hysteria and rage. The family is fragmented, and all the kids are placed in custody. The father is threatened with disgrace and imprisonment. The girl is blamed for causing the whole mess, and everyone seems to treat her like a freak. She is interrogated about all the tawdry details and encouraged to incriminate her father, yet the father remains unchallenged, remaining at home in the security of the family. She is held in custody, with no hope of returning home if the dependency petition is sustained.

The message from the mother is very clear, often explicit: "Why do you insist on telling those awful stories about your father? If you send him to prison we won't be a family anymore. We'll end up on welfare, with no place to stay. Is that what *you* want to do to us?"

Once again, the child bears the responsibility of either preserving or destroying the family. The role reversal continues, with the "bad" choice to tell the truth or the "good" choice to capitulate and restore a lie for the sake of the family.

Unless there is special support for the child and immediate intervention to force responsibility on the father, the girl will follow the "normal" course and retract her complaint. The girl "admits" she made up the story: "I was awful mad at my dad for punishing me. He hit me and said I could never see my boyfriend again. I've been really bad for years and nothing seems to keep me from getting into trouble. Dad had plenty of reason to be mad at me. But I got real mad and just had to find some way of getting out of that place. So I made up this story about him fooling around with me and everything. I didn't mean to get everyone in so much trouble."

This simple lie carries more credibility than the most explicit claims of incestuous entrapment. It confirms adult expectations that children can't be trusted. It restores the precarious equilibrium of the family. The children learn not to complain. The adults learn not to listen. And the authorities learn not to believe rebellious children who try to use their sexual power to destroy well-meaning parents. Case closed.

PSYCHODYNAMIC DETERRENTS TO RECOGNITION

Now that some of the myths and enigmas of sexual abuse have been discussed, it is worth repeating Suzanne Sgroi's cardinal rule of recognition: "Recognition of sexual molestation of a child is entirely dependent on the individual's inherent willingness to entertain the possibility that the condition may exist" (1975, p. 20). It is important also to consider the companion statement from Dr. Sgroi: "Unfortunately, willingness to consider the diagnosis of suspected child molestation seems to vary in inverse proportion to the individual's level of training" (1975, p. 20). Behavioral scientists are schooled to be skeptical of children's accounts of sexual activity. Enlightenment in the complexities of psychosexual development and oedipal psychodynamics tends to create a bias toward defining a fantasy basis rather than reality when evaluating a child's memories of sexual experiences with caring adults. This bias follows the precedent set by Freud himself in confronting the dilemma of fantastic-sounding complaints. As Freud wrote in 1933, "Almost all my women patients told me that they had been seduced by their father. I was driven to recognize in the end that those reports were untrue and so came to understand that the hysterical symptoms were derived from fantasy and not from real occurrences" (p. 584).

As early as 1893, Joseph Breuer and his pupil, Sigmund Freud, published in *Studies on Hysteria* the first reported observation that childhood sexual trauma could lead to symptoms of hysteria. As Freud developed his techniques of psychoanalysis, he was troubled by the persistent implications of sexual trauma he found in each of his patients with hysteria. His conclusion that childhood seduction was the basis for hysteria led to scathing criticism from both of his teachers, Charcot and Breuer, as well as most of his other colleagues in the *Doktorenkollegium*. The troubling implications of widespread parent-child sexuality seem to have driven Breuer from psychology back into the safer, more socially acceptable study of pulmonary physiology (Peters, 1976). Freud sought to minimize professional outrage on behalf of respectable fathers by documenting less controversial relationships. He acknowledged 30 years later that two of the patients described in *Studies on Hysteria* had been seduced not by their uncles, as originally described, but by their fathers (Peters, 1976). Outrage increased, however, in response to Freud's determined assertion of his seduction theory in *The Aetiology of Hysteria* (1896), in which he concluded: "I therefore put forward the thesis that at the bottom of every case of hysteria there are *one or more occurrences of premature sexual experiences,* occurrences which belong to the earliest years of childhood" (p. 203).

While Freud must have been distressed by his colleagues' rejection of the seduction theory, he was also troubled personally by the potential accusation of innocent fathers. Following his own father's death in October, 1896, Freud wrote to his friend and confidant, Wilhelm Fliess, that he was unexpectedly troubled and distracted by his father's death and by a number of dreams and associated memories relating to his own early sexual feelings. He discovered from self-analysis the reality of early childhood sexuality, of desires for his mother, hatred of his father, and fear of reprisals from his father. He interpreted his guilt over his father's death as a reflection of an unconscious death wish. As he became aware of ambivalence toward fathers, he began to understand his uncertainty over the role of fathers as seducers of children. On February 11, 1897, he wrote to Fliess that he had been alarmed by the number of fathers named by his patients as molesters, and that he had come to fear, through the presence of hysterical symptoms in his sisters, that even his own father had been incriminated (Jones, 1961, p. 211). When he dreamed about his daughter, Mathilda, he took it to mean he was trying too hard to blame fathers as universally incestuous. As he wrote to Fliess on May 31, 1897, "Not long ago I dreamt that I was feeling over-affectionately towards Mathilda, but her name was 'Hella'. . . . She had a passion for the mythology of ancient Hellas and naturally regards all Hellenes as heroes. The dream, of course, fulfills my wish to pin down a father as the originator of neurosis and put an end to my persistent doubts" (Bonaparte, Freud, and Kris, 1954, pp. 206-207). Freud included in the same letter his observation that death wishes against parents were an integral part of neurosis, with men directing their hostility against their fathers and women against their mothers.

Through self-analysis Freud moved from the belief that female children are damaged by adult seduction and that large numbers of fathers must be inherently incestuous to the recognition that all children (male and female) have sexual desires for a parent, leading to feelings of guilt, jealousy, and unconscious death wishes against the other parent. Neurosis need not be attributed to an abusive parent nor limited to individuals who had been actually abused; all children are subject to maladjustments arising from their inability to cope with the psychic consequences of their own perverse sexual needs and vengeful fantasies.

Within a few months he was able to repudiate his seduction theory and to express a feeling of triumph in leaving its uncertainties behind. On September 21, he wrote to Fliess:

> Let me tell you straight away the great secret which has been slowly dawning on me in recent months. I no longer believe in my neurotica. . . . I shall start at the beginning and tell you the whole story of how the reasons for rejecting it arose. The first group of factors were the continual disappointment of my attempts to bring my analysis to a real conclusion, the running away of people who for a time had seemed my most favorably inclined patients, the lack of the complete success on which I had counted, and the possibility of explaining my partial success in other familiar ways. Then there was the astonishing thing that in every case . . . blame was laid on perverse acts by the father, and the realisation of the unexpected frequency of hysteria, in every case of which the same applied, though it was hardly credible that perverted acts against children were so general. . . . Thirdly, there was the definite realisation that there is no 'indication of reality' in the unconscious, so that it is impossible to distinguish between truth and emotionally-charged fiction. (This leaves open the possible explanation that sexual phantasy regularly makes use of the theme of parents) (Bonaparte, Freud, and Kris, 1954, pp. 215-217).

Freud had by now assembled the basic components for the unifying theory of psychoneurosis, based on infantile sexuality and incestuous fantasies, which was to become known as the Oedipus complex. On October 15, 1897 he wrote to Fliess:

> I have found love for the mother and jealousy of the father in my own case too and now believe it to be a general phenomenon of early child-hood. . . . If that is the case the gripping power of Oedipus Rex . . . becomes intelligible, and one can understand why later dramas were such failures. . . . The Greek myth seizes on a compulsion which everyone recognizes because he has felt traces of it in himself. Every member of the audience was once a budding oedipus in phantasy, and his dream-fulfillment played out in reality causes everyone to recoil in horror, with the full measure of repression which separates his infantile from his present state (Bonaparte, Freud, and Kris, pp. 223-224).

After *The Aetiology of Hysteria* in 1896, Freud never advanced any aspect of the seduction theory again, except to apologize in footnotes to later editions for his earlier naiveté in accepting his patients' reports at face value. In a 1924 footnote to *The Aetiology of Hysteria* he explains:

> This section is dominated by an error which I have since repeatedly acknowledged and corrected. At that time I was not yet able to distinguish between my patients' phantasies about their childhood years and their real recollections. As a result I attributed to the aetiological factor of seduction a significance and universality which it does not possess (Freud, 1896 (1924), p. 168).

The Oedpius complex offered not only the attraction of universality, it served also as a fortuitous, adult-reassuring alternative to the seduction theory. Children, not their fathers, were responsible for the allegations of sexual abuse. It was the perverse needs of the child that scapegoated adults with undeserved accusations. Finally, whatever children (or adults) chose to say about sexual experiences with their parents, it must be assumed to be wishful fantasy unless proven otherwise.

Freud's early discovery was therefore an idea ahead of its time. Neither Freud nor the adult-protective world of that time was ready to explore or to validate the implications of the seduction theory. Not only was the theory discredited. Worse than that, the adult-protective reaction served to discourage and delay any subsequent reappraisal of that discovery. Freud's precocious, outrageous early speculation led him and many of his followers to arm themselves with a dogma of disbelief. The messenger of incest risks provoking not only ordinary, common-sense denial, but also inviting charges of heresy among the most highly trained and sophisticated professionals.

Joseph Peters combined his experience as director of the Sex Offender and Rape Victim Center, Philadelphia General Hospital, with his sensitivity as a practicing psychoanalyst to propose a new look at Freud's shift from the seduction theory to the Oedipus complex. In a paper written in 1976, he reviewed the impact of that shift on psychiatric thought:

> After 1924 the notion that hysterical symptoms were based upon actual events, real sexual assaults upon children, fell increasingly out of favor. Psychoanalysts abandoned the search for a distinction between actual childhood sexual trauma and children's fantasies. In the Freudian theory of psychoneurosis, the fantasies became as important as real events. Since Freud's thinking developed in this way, his earlier followers were relieved from facing the fact that patients sometimes had been real victims of sexual assault. . . . It is my thesis that both cultural and personal factors combined to cause everyone, including Freud himself at times, to welcome the idea that reports of childhood sexual victimization could be regarded as fantasies. This position relieved the guilt of adults. In my opinion, both Freud and his followers oversubscribed to the theory of childhood fantasy and overlooked incidents of actual sexual victimization in childhood (Peters, 1976, p. 401).

> In their aversion to what are often repulsive details, psychotherapists allowed and continue to allow their patients to repress emotionally significant, pathogenic factors. . . . In addition, it is important to note that because the reported offender was frequently the patient's own father, in order to avoid the fact of incest, my colleagues seized upon the easier assumption that the occurrences were oedipal fantasies (p. 402).

> Relegating these traumas to the imagination may divert treatment into a prolonged unraveling of natural developmental processes in which fantasy is a component. Furthermore, unsuccessful psychotherapeutic evaluation opens the way for prescribing . . . antipsychotic drugs and electroshock. The treatment may compound the patient's original psychologic problems. Ascribing these events to psychological fantasy may be easier and more interesting for the therapist, but it may also be counterproductive for the most efficient resolution of symptoms (pp. 407–408).

> An immediate supportive response by parents, criminal justice personnel, doctors and nurses is crucial to preserve the emotional integrity of the child. Particularly when the offender is a member of the family, care must be taken by service personnel to insure that the child's needs are put first (Peters, 1976, p. 421).

Florence Rush, writing from a feminist perspective with scholarly documentation from the psychoanalytic literature, challenges Freud's shift to the Oedipus complex, especially in the concepts of penis envy and the universal wish of little girls to possess their father's penis.

> As he approached the source of the neurosis, and evolved the now-famous Oedipal complex, Freud freely applied his particularly personal discovery to everybody, to all cultures, and to females as well as males (Rush, 1977, p. 37).

The seduction theory maintained that hysteria was a neurosis caused by sexual assault, and it incriminated incestuous fathers, while the Oedipal theory insisted the seduction was a fantasy, an invention, not a fact—and it incriminated daughters. . . . However, one must remember that when Freud arrived at the seduction theory, he did so by listening carefully and intently to his female patients; when he arrived at his Oedipal theory, he did so by listening carefully and intently to himself. . . . Freud therefore cautioned the world never to overestimate the importance of seduction and the world listened to Freud and paid little heed to the sexual abuse of children (p. 39).

The reason is illogical, It categorically assigns a real experience to fantasy, or harmless reality at best, while the known offender—the one concrete reality—is ignored. With reality sacrificed to a nebulous unconscious, the little girl has no recourse. She is trapped within a web of adult conjecture and it is offered not protection, but treatment for some speculative ailment, while the offender—Uncle Willie, the grocery clerk, the dentist, or the child's father—is permitted further to indulge his predilection for little girls. The child's experience is as terrifying as the worst horror of a Kafkesque nightmare: her story is not believed, she is declared ill, and, worse, she is left at the mercy and the 'benevolence' of psychiatrically oriented 'child experts' (p. 40).

It is indeed strange how psychology is used not to help, but to trap and ensnare the female. The myth of consent—that is, the female desire to get a man, to have a penis—is used to explain victim participation and therefore accepts as inevitable the sexual abuse of children. The tragedy is that this myth is believed and that so often the victims are punished. Once a child has been raped or molested, no matter how impressive the psychological nomenclature describing her plight or how sophisticated her caretakers, the little girl is an outcast, a nymphomaniac, a whore (p. 41).

The little girl, then, with her innate passion for a penis, is—as in Christian doctrine—the temptress Eve, and, if she is violated, the nature of her sexuality renders her culpable. Any attempt on the part of the family to expose the violator also exposes her own alleged innate sexual motives and shames her more than the offender; concealment is her only recourse. The dilemma of sexual abuse of children has provided a system of fullproof emotional blackmail; if the victim incriminates the abuser, she also incriminates herself. The sexual abuse of the child is therefore the best-kept secret in the world (Rush, 1977, p. 45).

There are many other factors, of course, besides psychoanalytic concepts that stigmatize the child victims, and many of them penalize the boy as well as the girl. Psychiatrists are likely to be offended by the angry edge in Ms. Rush's attack on "child experts." The quotations from her thoughtful and thought-provoking article, "The Freudian Cover-Up" are included here not to alienate mental health specialists nor to widen the feminist-Freudian schizm, but to illustrate two current clinical realities. First, rape-crisis services, battered-women's shelters, incest-survivors' groups and other feminist-oriented resources that do active case finding in sexual abuse typically will not refer clients to psychoanalytically oriented treatment centers. A potentially vital link in the hospital-community network is broken unless there can be active efforts to develop shared priorities and values. Second, while not all mental health specialists stigmatize victims with prejudicial interpretations and labels, many do. Sexual abuse treatment networks have to search for psychiatrists who can "believe in" child sexual abuse and who are also willing to appear in court to help offset the inevitable "child fantasy" or "seductive child" expert opinion provided by the defense.

Mothers who leave a sexually abusive husband may go bankrupt trying to buy testimony that will challenge the father's demands for child custody. If a woman allows sexual abuse to occur under her roof, she is accused for setting up the abuse. If she separates with her children, she is accused of inventing prejudicial stories to block her estranged husband's legitimate access to his children. Clinical evaluation of the disputing parties and the children provides the major evidence in such suits, and the "objective" evaluation almost invariably faults the woman. The man is evaluated as normal if he is sufficiently self-assured and if he confides no more conflicted material than the average unemotional, well-defended male. The woman is evaluated as within normal limits, but with marked anxieties in the areas of sexuality. Projective testing is characterized by themes of loss of security, fear of attack, and of jeopardy and rescue for children. The woman typically will be quite candid in discussing marital discord, sexual incompatibility, and childhood family conflicts—all of which go to court as evidence of instability and punitive vested interest. The keystone of the argument is the evaluation of the child. The younger the child; the more sensitive the mother has been in picking up subliminal clues to abuse; and the more accommodated the child has become in trying to heal the split between the parents, the more ineffectual the examination will be. The verbal, expressive child will be interpreted as fantasizing or as reflecting the anxiety and coaching of the mother. The blocked or concealing child will be written off as either untouched or noncontributory. It is not unusual to read evaluations of children in which no direct questions were asked relating to sexual material in the belief that such questioning would be either punitive and intrusive or might fuel additional fantasy.

The following report was written by a psychiatrist evaluating the father in such a dispute. The father was suing for full custody of his 3-year-old son and 14-month-old daughter on the charge that his estranged wife was mentally unfit to care for the children. He alleged that his wife had fabricated charges against him in order to deprive him of custody: "She fabricated these charges against me; so I think she's very emotionally disturbed."

The mother had sought protective service intervention and psychiatric help for the boy, reporting he had complained of mutual masturbation and mutual oral intercourse while on visits with his father. According to the mother, the child had also demonstrated to her how his father had taught him to bend over, grasping his ankles, while his father inserted his finger and attempted to put his penis in the child's "tushy hole." She also described threats reported by the child that his father would go away and never see him again if the child told his mother. The mother had recorded in diary form a series of hints and increasingly specific complaints made by the boy beginning about a month after the parents separated. She sought protective service intervention within two weeks of the first hint that the father might have handled the child's penis, saying that at first she had been afraid to believe such a thing could be true.

Most of the psychiatric evaluation of the father is devoted to extended verbatim quotations of the man's complaints about his wife. Out of seven pages of single-spaced material, there is a six-line summary of sexual history: "He first had sexual relations in his early 20's; never engaged in any perverse homosexual practices, and had a good sexual relationship with first wife before and during marriage. His second wife was very slow to arouse, but enjoyed sexual relations and usually had climaxes."

The diagnostic opinion says, in effect, that a man who presents so well in clinical evaluations could not molest such a small child, or if he did molest a child it was the wife's fault:

> Defendant/subject is not mentally disordered, and there is no evidence from his history or clinical examination that he is sexually perverse or tends to pedophilia.
>
> He has a somewhat aggressive and rigid manner, with relatively little empathy expressed in this procedure—but much of his defensiveness and criticism of his wife are appropriate to the circumstances in which his wife's charges have placed him and to other behavior on her part which he described.

His religiosity, character, history, record, concern for children's welfare, and the tender age of alleged victim make the charges against him most unlikely to be based on facts of his behavior.

If committed, offense acts were precipitated by loneliness, anger at wife, and intimate circumstances—very unlikely to be repeated. He is not a danger, not in need of hospital treatment, and not a 'mentally disordered sex offender.'

Save for the charges, there appears no reason subject is unfit for child custody; and to the degree his description of his wife's behavior is accurate, her emotional stability is questionable, and if her charges are found to be fabricated, she is very unstable and unreliable, and reveals her disregard for the children's need for contact with both parents.

This report is not an isolated aberration: two subsequent evaluations, one by a clinical psychologist and another by a court-appointed psychiatrist, have been similarly prejudiced against the mother's complaints. The third examiner was most outspoken in condemning the "highly emotional" and "naive" reactions of those who reported child abuse:

I must say the naivete and unprofessionalism of this report shocked me. Sheldon told her (the play therapist) that his father put his penis in Sheldon's mouth and his thumb up his anus. . . . I must comment that what is so remarkable and psychiatrically naive is that what Sheldon was telling (the therapist) was *undoubtedly* a fantasy. Not only is it common psychiatric knowledge that children of all ages, and especially children from the ages of 3 to 5, engage in quite intensive sexual fantasies about their own and parents bodies but also fantasize any manner of sexuality that would be considered "perverse" by adults. I am not saying that I can claim with certainty that Sheldon is not reporting real events, but the distinction between reality and fantasy is not clear. . . . However, I am saying that *"perverse" sexual fantasies are to be expected at this age* and if a child did not have some of them, that would be considered an abnormality. . . . They are the fantasies of a child who is anxious about the affectional bonds with both his parents and is perhaps sexually overstimulated unconsciously by both of them, although *most certainly* by the mother, who is quite sexually preoccupied. What is also clear is that *Sheldon is quite turned on by women.* And although some homosexual urges towards his father are also obviously present in his fantasies, we see that even these fantasies come up only in situations where *he is being seductive* to women. An oedipus complex at this age with sexual longings primarily for the mother but also the father has been reported by psychoanalysts from the turn of the century and it shocks me that such an elementary piece of behavioral data is ignored. . . . When Sheldon reports to his grandmother about sexual activity between him and his father, this is brought up in the context and follows trying to *seduce* his grandmother into taking a bath with him. Later *he has her* examine his penis and he gets an erection in the process. In the long note that (the mother) wrote on the police report at initial contact, she gives a similar context. 'Sheldon tells me that he has to go to bed in my room' (after reporting sleeping with his father on the prior visit). At this point (the mother) asked Sheldon rather directly what is so special about going to bed with his father and Sheldon, who is *undoubtedly* still thinking about going to bed with his mother, describes the things that can be done in bed. . . . Later on (the mother) says "On April 8, 1980 I was giving Sheldon his bath. I showed him how to retract his foreskin and wash his penis. He said no, my dad says you do it slow and demonstrates rubbing very slowly across the head of the penis." *Clearly* he is showing his mother what *he wants from her* and how he wants her to do it. . . . There is also abundant other data that these are fantasies that we are involved with, e.g. the theme of castration by his father. This particular anxiety is part of the growing oedipal attachment to the mother, and the fantasy that the father is going to cut off his penis *is as predictable as the rising of the sun.*

The italics in the quotation above are added to emphasize the imperative terms used to demand acceptance of a theoretical, oedipal, mother-stimulating and child-seductive explanation for the reported sexual material. Among 15 single-spaced pages of very thoughtful and careful discussion, it is only when attacking the "emotional" involvement of those who intervened on behalf of the child's complaints that prejudicial language was used.

Did the father molest the child? It is impossible to know or to predict on theoretical or statistical grounds. But the child and a passionately protective parent must have some right to literal credibility. It is at least as logical to believe that a child overstimulated by his father would try to test the meaning of his experiences through reenactment with maternal figures as that he fantasized experiences with his father out of projected lust for his mother. And if a child is searching for a way to communicate confusing sexual experiences, wouldn't the bathtub be a good place to start, in the midst of touching by a safer, more trusted figure? It is difficult to imagine what a child might say or enact regarding an actual sexual molestation by a parent demanding secrecy and threatening bodily harm that would not be translated into oedipal terms. And how can a mother be responsive to a child's sexual distress without being labeled as sexually preoccupied or seductive? And what complaints should a therapist accept as real without being condemned as naive and unprofessional? Florence Rush has a point.

Why should a chapter on clinical recognition and management of sexual abuse be so burdened by the polemics of legal, domestic, and ideological disputes, with so much emphasis on reports and testimony to the courts? The answer is simple and vital: advocacy for the victim is the most basic and the most challenging function any physician can perform in the area of child sexual abuse. Any physician who must remain adult-protective, male-protective, or self-protective, and any physician who cannot communicate accurately and fairly with protective agencies can be only obstructive to the needs of the victim.

CLINICAL RECOGNITION OF SEXUAL ABUSE

Once the clinician is sensitive to the realities and patterns of sexual abuse, and when there is no longer a reluctance to ask the questions and to accept the answers, sexual abuse leaps to attention with bewildering frequency. Beyond the intangibles of increased sensitivity to subliminal clues, the cardinal tool for clinical recognition is the ability to ask a simple, direct question without embarrassment or fear in *every* pediatric examination. The question is not "Have you ever been sexually molested?" or "Has anyone ever molested you?"—both of which inspire fear and invite a hasty denial. A more congenial, more universal question might be something like, "How often do you feel icky or uncomfortable from the way someone touches you or plays with you?" or, "Do you know any grown-ups who play secret games with children's bodies?" or, "How many grown-ups and relatives do you really feel safe with?"

If a child seems comfortable or naively confused with the implications of such questions, there is opportunity for a preventive educational follow-up: "You're very lucky if you've never had to feel scared or uncomfortable with grown-ups. Some grown-ups, even daddies or mommies or other relatives, act like bullies sometimes and make children play with their bodies or they handle children's bodies in ways that don't feel right. Kids are usually afraid to complain or tell anyone, so they think they have to keep secrets and feel bad. If anything like that ever happened to you, I hope you'd tell me and give me a chance to help you. I promise I would understand and be on your side. I don't want any child to have to feel alone or afraid."

If there are symptoms of emotional distress or disturbed behavior indicating possible sexual abuse (see Table 10-1), questions should be more explicit and should be reinforced in each successive visit. When clinical suspicion merits such concern, questions should be deliberately leading and preceded by expressions of understanding and empathy to counteract the predictable distress and fear, as well as to address the typical feelings of isolation and guilt: "Most of the girls I see with this kind of upset are afraid to talk about something very secret that is happening to them. Some grown-up, like their uncle or father or some special

TABLE 10-1 INDICATORS OF SEXUAL ABUSE

A. Presumptive Indicators of Sexual Abuse
  1. Direct reports from children. False reports from young children are relatively rare; concealment is much more the rule. Adolescents may rarely express authority conflicts through distorted or exaggerated complaints, but each such complaint should be sensitively evaluated
  2. Pregnancy. Rule out premature but peer-appropriate sexual activity
  3. Prepubescent venereal disease
  4. Genital or rectal trauma. Remember that most sexual abuse is seductive rather than coercive and that the approach to small children may be nongenital. The presence or absence of a hymen is nonspecific to sexual abuse

B. Possible Indicators
  1. Precocious sexual interest or preoccupation
  2. Indiscreet masturbatory activity
  3. Genital inflammation or discharge. More often masturbatory or foreign body than abusive. The three items above most often indicate a sexually stimulating environment or a sexually permissive environment, which may not be deliberately abusive nor intrusive
  4. Apparent pain in sitting or walking. Be alert for evasive or illogical explanations. Encourage physical examination

C. Behavioral and Clinical Associations: Nonspecific
  1. Social withdrawal and isolation
  2. Underachievement, distraction, and "daydreaming"
  3. Indications of any parental child abuse or neglect
  4. Fear and distrust of authorities
  5. Identification with authorities. Too-willing acquiescence to adult demands may represent a conditioned response to parental intrusion and a high vulnerability to adult exploitation
  6. Negative self-esteem, depression, suicidal behavior, substance abuse
  7. Somatic complaints: abdominal or pelvic pain, nausea, vomiting, anorexia, dysphagia, headache
  8. Dissociative states, hysterical phenomena, multiple personality.
  9. Atypical seizures
  10. Sleep disorders
  11. Normal, peer-appropriate behavior and achievement. Remember that many children will carefully conceal any sign of sexual victimization. Attempts at compensation may even lead to overachievement, extraordinary social skills, and model behavior

NOTE: This outline is intended only as a superficial inventory of signs of potential sexual abuse as they might be observed by a teacher, school nurse, parent, or physician. The list is neither exhaustive nor specific. No attempt is made to correlate these isolated signs with the clinical and descriptive information needed for further evaluation, investigation, diagnosis, and management of sexual problems in children. This outline should be used only in conjunction with study and professional consultation in sexual problems. Any firm suspicion of sexual abuse must by law be reported to the appropriate authorities.

friend, has taught them to be sexual with them. The child usually feels all alone and afraid nobody can help or understand. Lots of times they think it's their fault, or they've been told terrible things would happen if they don't keep it a secret. They don't know that men with that kind of problem need help to stop getting sexual with little kids. And they don't know that lots of kids have found help by getting someone else to stop it. I can understand things like that; it's my job. And I know other people who have special jobs just to protect kids and to help their families to take care of them. Anyway, that's the way it was with other kids, and they're glad they didn't keep the secret any longer. I wonder if something like that has been happening to you?"

Acknowledgment may be tentative or it may come pouring out like a flood. In any case, whoever is taking the history should be rewarding and supporting of disclosure. An outstretched hand or an offered embrace will go a long way to offset the child's fear that she is making herself reprehensible through the disclosure. In general, a girl will be more comfortable with a female examiner. More important than gender, though, is the level of comfort and experience reflected by the clinician.

It should be understood that the more prevalent forms of sexual abuse involve little physical trauma and no visible tissue damage. A careful and well-documented physical is all the more important. The child will be reassured by the doctor who can say, "I've checked you over very thoroughly inside and out, and there's no sign of any damage or any kind of change in your body. Once you get help to get over the bad feelings, you'll be perfectly OK again. You don't have to worry that there's anything about your experience that shows."

The patient's chart becomes crucial evidence in subsequent court actions. The victim's statements to a clinician during the distress of initial disclosure may be acceptable as *prima-facie* evidence, despite later distortions or retractions. Statements outside of clinical evaluation, whether to parents or police officers, are regarded only as hearsay. The child's welfare is betrayed by the offhand jargon typical of so many charts: "Child seen because of alleged sexual abuse. P.E. w.n.l. External genitalia o. Pelvic deferred. No indication of sexual activity." With explicit documentation of the child's complaints, specific description of the genital exam, and a statement that the sexual activity described would normally leave no signs of trauma, the clinical evaluation speaks for the child. As written here, the exam will be used to dispute the child's claims.

There should be a protocol for adequate evaluation and documentation of each child presenting with indications of sexual abuse. All clerical, nursing, social work, and medical personnel who have contact with children should be trained in appropriate response and coordination of roles for the support of the child and the family. The protocols of the Sexual Assault Center at Harborview Medical Center, University of Washington School of Medicine, Seattle (Appendix) are a good example of the advantages inherent in preplanning and coordination of specialized services for victims of sexual abuse. The protocols also illustrate the importance of proper collection and handling of laboratory specimens indicated both for diagnosis and for legal documentation.

Recognition of sexual abuse in males is especially difficult. Clinical sensitivity must be acute, since boys are even less likely than girls to volunteer sexual information. Of the victimized boys in Finkelhor's sample (1979a) only about one-fourth told anyone. Victimized boys tend to fall into two rather polarized categories: (1) forcible, often physically traumatic sexual assault, and (2) careful, premeditated sexualization of an ongoing, affectionate pedophilic relationship. The traumatized boy will avoid disclosure for fear of retaliation and from a sense of unmanliness and shame at being weak and helpless. The partner to affectionate seduction will be protective and idealistically defensive of the relationship. Boys often feel threatened by the stigma and fear of homosexuality attached to their involvement with a male. Counterphobic denial and exaggerated macho behavior with girls may give clues to occult victimization.

TREATMENT OF SEXUAL ABUSE

Any concept of treatment of sexual abuse must include a variety of resources and services beyond those ordinarily available to a hospital or medical clinic setting. The medical model is not incapable of expanding into multimodal services, but without a somewhat radical realignment of priorities there is a tendency to undervalue the child-protective, law enforcement, parental support, and child-reparenting aspects vital to a comprehensive program. A hospital-based or office model built on patient-initiated, voluntary requests for professional services at scheduled intervals cannot meet the needs of children who are alienated from the advocacy of their parents nor the frustrations of parents who cannot be assumed to be responsible for their children. The success of the physician and any paramedical specialist will be dependent on the ability to develop an innovative style of interagency outreach and the willingness to share therapeutic roles with an extended network of community services.

At least three cherished traditions of American medicine are challenged by the interagency model:

1. *Authority.* The physician may have relatively less experience, contact, and salient data than other investigators in a given case. Clinical impressions may be overruled by police evidence or protective service findings. Or conclusive medical evidence may be ignored in court decisions. Clinicians accustomed to having the ultimate authority in management decisions will be aliented and distrustful in a relatively subordinate role.

2. *Fee for Service.*   The private practitioner may feel in competition with publicly funded, philanthropic, or voluntary self-help aspects of an integrated program. Turf disputes and chauvinistic defensiveness on both sides of the fee barrier may exploit clients to distrust the quality of free services on one hand or the sincerity of paid services on the other.

3. *Sanctuary.*   The physician shares with the priest and the attorney the carefully guarded power of confidentiality. The physician-patient relationship offers the implicit guarantee that a person in need of care will not be exposed to social or political intervention. Child abuse reporting laws are a specific and sometimes problematic exception to privileged communication. The physician finds neither precedent nor comfort in informing police and social agencies of suspected child abuse, especially when reporting violates the expressed wish of the child and parents for a confidential, clinical resolution of their "family adjustment problem." It is often tempting to avoid reporting to spare both family and physician the anxiety and uncertainties of a compromise in clinical control. Yet the success of coordinated programs contrasts sharply with the high dropout rate and limited disclosure of families who are offered clinical sanctuary (Summit, 1978). Like it or not, the physician is subject to both criminal and civil liability if reporting mandates are ignored.

Design and coordination of an effective sexual abuse treatment program requires experiential training, community organization, and locally adaptive adjustments, all of which lie beyond the scope of this chapter. In addition, the available models and concepts of sexual abuse treatment are expanding so rapidly that no one publication can give a really timely or comprehensive appraisal of the immediate state of the art. Several excellent texts, articles, and training programs are available. *Sexual Assault of Children and Adolescents* (Burgess, Groth, and Holmstrom, 1978), Giarretto's (1976) chapter in Helfer and Kempe, *Sexually Victimized Children* (Finkelhor, 1979a), and *Dealing with Sexual Child Abuse*, Vol. 2, published by The National Committee for Prevention of Child Abuse (1978), are essential references. Textbooks should be supplemented by a comprehensive review of the current professional literature in the subject categories of child abuse, sexual abuse, incest, victimization, pedophilia, and sexual offenses. The National Center on Child Abuse and Neglect funds several regional training programs in sexual abuse management, including currently the Parents United model in Santa Clara County, California, and the Sexual Assault Center in Seattle. Information on available programs can be obtained by writing The National Center on Child Abuse and Neglect, Department of Health and Human Services, P.O. Box 1182, Washington DC 20013.

Any program treating sexual abuse should be closely linked with other community programs related to child abuse, child development, and parent education. Lessons learned in dealing with abusive and neglectful parents provide new understanding of the essentials of positive parenting. The ideals of empathic parenting, constructive discipline, and enhancement of self-esteem are best learned by abusive parents in association with other families with less abusive backgrounds.

Community councils on child abuse or family violence offer an exciting forum for shared development and support of services for children. Anyone developing a sexual abuse treatment program should work to develop such a council or to support an existing network. An excellent training film, "Child Abuse, A Chain to be Broken," describes the purposes and potentials of community networking.

KEY ELEMENTS IN SPECIALTY TREATMENT PROGRAMS

Sexually abusive families have a number of special needs that must be met in the course of intervention and treatment. These factors are more fully discussed elsewhere (Summit, 1978) and will be explored here as general principles.

Child Protection

The greatest single failure of traditional treatment and counseling approaches when applied to child abuse is the continued reliance on the parents for child advocacy. The therapist who depends on the motivation of conflicted parents to keep appointments and to verbalize humiliating parent-child identity struggles will conclude that abusive families are untreatable. And the therapist who monitors the welfare of the child only through office descriptions from the parent is depending on the fox to look after the hen house. It must be assumed that the parents begin treatment in an inverted role, depending on children to meet their needs, and that they will be both fearful and jealous of protective attention directed to the child. Just as the parent denies and conceals any ongoing abuses, the child continues to seek security and approval by shielding the parent from discovery. In many cases the mother will be unquestionably supportive and protective of her child. In other cases the mother will require reassurance and reinforcement that the child is telling the truth and that the child is not to blame for the initiation of the sexual behavior.

Many sexually abused children will require initial separation from both parents. Eventual reunification must be carefully monitored to protect the child from slipping back into the inverted role of subordinating personal welfare to the needs of the parent. Children will typically echo their mother's urgent wish to patch together an early return of the father, despite their own unexpressed fears and feelings of betrayal. The child's therapist must take the lead in translating ambivalent fears and tentative complaints into protective demands. It is unfair to leave to the child the choice of whether to report that the father is back home, in violation of a court order, or that she feels sexually threatened by the way he holds, tickles, teases, or wrestles with her. We do our child patients no favors by abdicating adult supervision too soon or by saddling the very young with the responsibility for their own survival.

Treatment staff working in conjunction with protective services and courts must advocate for the child's comfort despite superficial treatment gains professed by the parents. The entire treatment team must be on guard against a strong societal and professional idealism that seeks to keep families together and to preserve adult authority at all costs.

This precaution is not meant to encourage another reactive excess: a tendency to punish parents by depriving them forever of any contact with their children. In both extremes the children serve as pawns in the self-protective or punitive skirmishes of adult-oriented systems. The therapist must decide whether to report new abuses, whether to report violations of court orders, and how soon to advocate for reconstitution of families. Those decisions must be based not on wishful thinking, therapeutic optimism, prejudicial conservatism, countertransference issues, programmatic convenience, or blind tradition. They must be based on a canny and realistic appraisal of what best speaks for the psychic integrity, autonomy, and identity of the child.

With experience, most therapists in specialty child abuse treatment programs develop comfort in discovering and reporting abusive trends as part of their advocacy for the parents as well as their protection of the child. The therapist achieves a new maturity in the process of reparenting an abusive parent. The therapist, like any effective parent, must be willing to carry the burden of defining limits and upholding discipline at the risk of being resented or considered unfair. The challenge for any therapist or parent is to define discipline in the context of growth and to apply any judgments and proscriptions of behavior upon a well-established foundation of caring and endorsement for the person.

Court Advocacy

Court intervention is an overwhelming fact of life for the sexually abusive family. Fear of criminal prosecution, public disgrace, and family disruption creates a survival panic that belittles all other treatment issues.

Therapists themselves may panic in the process of identification with their patients. They may express distrust of shelter care facilities and try to sequester children from protective custody. Or they may feel that child-abusive behavior is an illness and that a parent should not be punished for uncontrollable impulses.

Or they may decide that the child must be protected at all costs from the agony of victim-witness testimony and cross-examination. Or the therapist may feel helpless and ineffectual or even fearful in attempting to deal with the court system. The list goes on and on with logical and self-comforting reasons to avoid dealing with court issues.

Avoidance of court involvement serves only to increase anxiety within the family and to leave courts ignorant of treatment and rehabilitation potentials. However unrealiable or capricious juvenile court decisions may seem and however punitive and damaging criminal actions may appear, the therapist must be willing to take an assertive role as an expert child advocate. While such advocacy generally speaks also for a favorable prognosis with cooperative parents, it may at times favor lifetime separation from recalcitrant offenders. Just as expert testimony speaks to the right of rehabilitation for selected incest offenders, it must also caution judges and prosecutors against unwarranted optimism for chronic sexual offenders. A treatment program with a good recovery record for incestuous fathers will be swamped with court referrals of overt and covert pedophiles unless admission criteria are repeatedly defined and strictly enforced.

While most incest treatment programs support appropriate child protection through the dependency court, there is a sharp division of opinion regarding criminal prosecution of incestuous fathers. Many programs encourage negotiation for treatment as an alternative to criminal action. There has been a trend to decriminalize parental violence in the hope of enhancing parental self-esteem and encouraging more voluntary participation in therapy. Advocates for decriminalization argue that the victim-perpetrator model of criminal prosecution is inappropriate for complex and interdependent family relationships. There is a well-founded fear that if fathers are encouraged to seek favorable consideration by admitting to charges of incest, they might be more severely punished than the treatment-resistent offender who flatly denies all charges. Finally, the cruel scapegoating and character assassination directed toward the victim-witness in an adversary proceeding are seen as more abusive to the child than the risks of nonprosecution.

While there is ample clinical experience to reinforce distrust of the criminal justice system as a therapeutic ally, I believe that the child's hope for maximum recovery is compromised by decriminalization. There is an enormous ethical contradiction in a position that tells a man it is a criminal offense to rape a child unless it is one of his own. And how can the child be assured that it was not her fault if we do not empower her to define a crime against her person? And how much is she worth as a person if such a crime is not charged? Of even more immediate consequence is the fact that most men will not submit to meaningful treatment and will not honestly examine their own culpability for incestuous abuse unless coerced through the fear of inescapable criminal reckoning. Punishment alone will do little for recovery. Treatment alone has little power to require painful disclosures and drastic changes in a man's balance of power.

The fear of court involvement that tends to resonate between therapists and patients can be decreased by a more pragmatic approach to the issues, a willingness to address the problems as part of therapy, and, especially, the assumption of more active therapeutic initiative and involvement within the court system. Staff should be trained, experienced, and confident in dealing with every aspect of the justice system. The treatment program must prepare child witnesses for their day in court and must help train prosecutors and judges to deal fairly and compassionately with children. These issues are explored in a paper, "Special Techniques for Child Witnesses" (Berliner and Stevens, 1979), and a training film, "*Double Jeopardy*," both developed by the Harborview Sexual Assault Center.

Outreach and Availability

Traditional systems of treatment assume that individuals will present themselves willingly and will confide freely whatever conflicts are troubling them. Office therapy also assumes that patients will be motivated to change their perceptions or behavior to decrease anxiety and to improve self-esteem. Traditional outpatient therapy depends on a patient's self-motivation to keep appointments and to take the risks of change. Individuals involved in sexual abuse tend to be desperately afraid of discovery, judgment, further stigmatization, and exposure. The sexual abuse itself tends to maintain adult control and a precarious sense of security that depends on secrecy and isolation. Giving up the behavior, losing control, exposing feelings, exploring adult dependency needs, and learning to trust others in a position of authority are all *anxiety-provoking* rather than reassuring experiences. This is especially true for those who have been consistently abused by parents and who were taught to accept blame and punishment for anything they do. For the self-hating victim of child abuse, whether current victim or grown-up father or mother, disclosure of abuse leads not to relief or insight but to further humiliation, self-blame, and self-punishment. A person conditioned to scapegoating and unreasonable punishment simply cannot accept that he or she will not be condemned and punished by insight and that the therapist, who seems so much like a parent, would not inevitably reject and punish anyone so patently offensive.

There is a sad irony in the reality that abused and abusive individuals so often must be coerced into therapy through threat of punishment. It is further ironic that so many victims will distrust and try to escape from anyone who offers the hope of a benevolent and nonpunitive reception. The therapist must anticipate these problems by giving unqualified reinforcement and support to each member of the conflict while drawing on outside coercion and control to maintain contact through the predictable stresses of engagement. The treatment interface must be *engaging*. The style of the counselors should be engaging, open, and

directly reassuring, even while requiring clearly defined limits on abusive behavior. A humanistic faith that any individual will seek his or her highest ideals
should be coupled with the pragmatic acceptance that anyone under threat will
fight to avoid exposure or change. Treatment develops as a dynamic progression
from fear, distrust, and hopeless avoidance to optimism, human acceptance, and
enthusiastic involvement. Missed appointments cannot be tolerated, but resched-
uling and unexpected crises must be accommodated without prejudice. If an
appointment is missed in the midst of a transference crisis, it is the responsibility
of the therapist to call and to reestablish contact. Whenever there is any risk of
child-abusive, self-mutilating, or suicidal behavior, there must be facility for
home visits and physical intervention by program staff. Engagement of reluctant,
self-defeating, potentially dangerous individuals cannot be accomplished by the
old "take two aspirins and call me in the morning" approach. If the program
presumes to understand and to care for the child-abusive family, it cannot
demand that the parents structure their needs and crises to serve the schedule
and style of the therapist.

In practice, most families will avoid making unreasonable or even reasonable
demands on the program. Early reinforcement of outreach and availability will
tend to encourage judgment and maturity in patients, allowing them to make the
best use of services to avoid explosive, untimely crisis demands.

Peer-Group Contact

Child abuse thrives on isolation and secrecy and it carries the seeds of its own
alienation and generational survival. The abused child learns to hide from discovery out of fear of further rejection and punishment and the related belief he
or she is inherently bad and deserving of contempt. The child grows up to
achieve a certain amount of adult acceptance and approval but with an inner
sense of counterfeit identity: "They accept me because they *don't know.* They
think I'm like them, but there's really nobody in the world like me. If they knew
how bad I am they'd hate me."

In accepting and in trying so hard to hide the stigma of abuse, the child defers
an awesome power to parents and other adults, as well as the potential to claim
some of that power after growing up into the role of parent. Abuse survivors
may be able to act as if they are comfortably adjusted while hiding enormous
and often poorly acknowledged self-hate and projections of destructive power
into their own children. When they find themselves resenting, exploiting, or
abusing their children, they may rationalize this as appropriate, in identification
with their own abusive parents. They can protect their image of the good, protective parent as well as protect themselves from memories of vulnerability by
overinvesting the parental role with righteousness and power. If this defensive

structure is threatened, either by compassion for the feelings of the child or by insight gained through treatment, the abused—now abusive—parent will seem to overreact into denial, panic, or flight with the discovery of the inner destructive power and the sense of being a monster (a word heard frequently in the productions of abused children and abusive parents).

Issues of smallness, helplessness, blame, guilt, pain, anger, disapproval, punishment, and rejection are so disproportionate that they tend to overwhelm the patient's transference toward an individual therapist, whatever the reality and style of that therapist. Whether male, female, gentle, directive, old, or young, the role and parental associations inherent in the psychotherapeutic process will provoke intense, defensive, often countertherapeutic parental transference in the abuse-scarred patient.

Psychoanalyst Leonard Shengold (1979, pp. 553-554) writes of the challenge to the psychotherapist in treating the victims of what he calls *soul murder*: consistent parental deprivation or abuse.

> Can we help them modify their misery on the basis of a human relationship (which is what we do as analysts) if they have never had and therefore perhaps never can have a decent human relationship?. . . . We require that our patients be capable of transference. Victims of soul murder may have very little that is positive to transfer. . . . We may be able to understand a good deal about how such people become what they are, but interpreting our knowledge may be of little help to them.

The compression of identity, self-worth, punishment, trust, and survival into the destructive parent-child relationship deprives the survivor of positive *mirroring*, either from the primary parent or from important others and peers. Since the survivor presents a counterfeit identity to others, any positive mirroring is perceived as ill-founded ("If they really knew they'd hate me"). Negative reactions, on the other hand, are accepted and amplified as genuine, especially from anyone with presumed knowledge and the parental power to penetrate the *as if* facade. Ordinary social support and professional attempts at reassurance are therefore not only poorly effective; they carry the threat of alienation and punishment whenever relationships become close or important.

Individual therapy, by itself, tends to be frustrating at best and countertherapeutic at worst. Trust and a capacity for positive transference can be built only over time and in conjunction with acceptance within a genuine peer group. The isolated, poorly disguised monster who is so distrustful and fearful of the image reflected by mainstream society discovers an unexpected acceptance and genuineness within the reflection of others who have shared the same stigmatizing experience. The others don't look like monsters and they don't seem to be repulsed by what they see in the newcomer. As the peer group makes it clear that nothing the newcomer can present is alien from the collective experience or capability, it becomes safe to drop the facade and to look intently into a new mirror.

While the metaphor of the mirror is too superficial and specifically visual to describe fully the complex benefits of a specialized peer group, it is part of the language of both group members and specialists in object relations. Within the affinity and the warm acceptance of the specialized peer group, the stigmatized victim "sees" and comes to feel that he or she is not uniquely cursed and that there is hope for genuine acceptance even without secrecy and self-deception. And the certain recognition that others are capable of surviving and of dealing directly with assaultive childhood experiences builds confidence that the evils of childhood can be confronted without humiliation or annihilation. *Seeing* others discuss and cope with child-abusive experience without humiliation or punishment allows the individual to challenge the self-fulfilling prophecy that *anyone* who knows would react with horror. Finally, the group can use its collective, emerging self-esteem to encourage individuals to present themselves to the outer society without shame and without expectations of prejudice.

Rather than preparing patients for group through individual counseling, group involvement should be used in most cases as the first resource for crisis intervention, with individual contact used as needed to coordinate overall treatment priorities and to deal with the consequences of the group experience. The initial use of the group helps to diffuse negative transference issues and to encourage a social model of resourcefulness rather than emphasizing dependency and possible regression within a more parental model of individual care. Intensive individual therapy, with deliberate exercises in regression and abreaction and with controlled enhancement of parental transference and reparenting, may be appropriate and necessary to repair the more seriously damaged survivors of soul murder. But such volatile and demanding techniques should be applied whenever possible on a foundation of preexisting peer-group identity and resources. Many who are not at first capable of trust or effective transference develop or recover enough ego strength through peer-group endorsement to take on the risk of intimacy in individual treatment and the challenge of finding a peer in the person of the psychotherapist.

The benefits of peer-group interaction apply also to the professional who works with the group. The leveling effects of the group as well as the prevailing candor and comfort initiate the therapist into the inside world of victim and victimizers and provide the therapist with an increased capacity for empathy. With the help of the peer group, the therapist is enabled to take on the risk of intimacy in individual treatment and the challenge of finding a peer in the person of the abused child and/or the abusive parent.

One of the great strengths of a specialty program for sexual abuse is the inherent potential for grouping of clients according to peer experience. Adult survivors; abusive parents; passively involved mates; adolescent offenders; and recent victims in preschool, latency-age, early-adolescent, and later-adolescent groupings all seem to benefit from peer-group contact and to achieve more rapid and more effective recovery than could be expected from individual therapy alone.

Self-Help

A logical extension of the strengths of the peer group is the encouragement of self-help. Parents United, Inc. is a modified self-help program that developed in conjunction with the Vanguard Child Sexual Abuse Treatment Project in Santa Clara County, California. Organized and incorporated by the parents themselves, Parents United uses both professional and peer counselors who lead specialized groups (orientation, men, women, couples, and women abused as children) as well as combining all participants in an opening and closing social-organizational gathering. Chapters also support separate groups for the children (Daughters and Sons United) and organize teams for telephone hot-line service, crisis outreach, shared residence (especially for fathers who agree to move away from home in deference to their children), agency outreach (advocating for more effective policies in the justice system, better support for treatment programs, etc.), and community education. Far from being counterprofessional or self-serving, the combined strength, energy, and conscience of so many participants freeing themselves from entrapment and stigma serve to endorse the importance of professional skills and the need for treatment system involvement in child-protective and law enforcement activities.

Remarkably, when incestuous fathers and stepfathers are empowered as a group to work toward preventing sexual abuse they are the first to encourage firm control and limits, including criminal investigation and prosecution. *The most effective deterrent to dismissed charges, adversary deadlocks, and child-witness humiliation is the power of a fathers' crisis intervention team to prevail on a peer to plead guilty or no contest and to accept compassionate sentencing and mandatory treatment rather than protesting his innocence.*

The immediate support of peers around issues of disclosure, separation, and rejection provides near-perfect protection against despondency, depression, and suicide. Fathers treated with hospitalization not infrequently leave the hospital only to commit suicide. Yet among thousands of families in California assisted by Parents United, not one father has been lost. Clinical intervention alone cannot extend support into the lonely hours when a father may be overwhelmed by loss, guilt, and hopelessness. Empathic fathers who have overcome such an experience and who feel a missionary kinship with the newly discovered offender will stay up through the night to provide companionship throughout the crisis.

The leadership and interaction of various advocacy positions within the self-help program helps to maintain internal balance and self-government without authoritarian demands or intervention from staff. Indignant, confident wives help strengthen those who would otherwise be hopelessly disillusioned or intimidated by their husbands' behavior. Women in general support one another against inappropriate or premature reconciliation with their husbands, as well as resisting a prevailing expectation of fathers that everyone should reward them with immediate expiation and loving reconciliation for their willingness to admit their fault. (The same narcissistic insensitivity that insulates fathers from the feelings of their children protects them also from appropriate responsibility to their wives: "Why do you keep bringing it up and punishing me? I already said I was sorry. What more do you want from me?") If husband and wife choose to reconcile, both may tend to defend against the impact of incest on their children, including a tendency to fault the child for reporting or for inviting "the incident" (ten years of ongoing rapacious, intimidating, and thoroughly obscene behavior can be trivialized and condensed into such a term). This tendency to seal over on the part of parental adults is offset by the presence in the chapter of another adult presence: that of the woman abused as a child who attends for her own recovery. These women may vary in age from newly emancipated later teens to senior citizens. Their apparent pain and their newly discovered determination to set their emotional records straight allow no room for trivialization of children's feelings or scapegoating of the children with any responsibility that belongs to the parents.

The chemistry of the large group interaction also fuels work in specialty subgroup and individual therapy. A mature survivor who is afraid to recognize anger toward her own father may be furious with another father she hears projecting blame on his child. Her passionate recognition that the child is blameless and unfairly treated can help her to respond to assurances in the survivor's group that she is now safe and secure enough to assign a similar blame and anger to her own father. And a father who is too rigidly defended to acknowledge his daughter's pain may be moved by the obvious, *adult-authenticated* distress expressed by the adult survivor to understand for the first time what his own daughter has experienced.

There are potential drawbacks, of course, to building self-help concepts into an integrated professional treatment system. Professionals may be distrustful or intimidated by the shift of power and responsibility to the patients. Therapists must be mature enough in their experience and professional identity to allow for such a diffusion of authority. Participation within the self-help style calls for informality and self-disclosures that may be antithetical to the training and comfort of the professional. Again, one must be quite secure to maintain balance in such an unaccustomed role.

At the same time, the staff must remain vigilant to protect the program against manipulative members who pretend to positions of authority. Would-be peer counselors who seek power in controlling others' decisions are a fairly obvious hazard. Charismatic sociopaths are a more difficult problem. The self-help approach tends to be self-leveling and endorsing of mainstream values as long as the fathers are dedicated to recovering age-appropriate sexual partners and as long as there has not been a lifetime rationalization of sexual intimidation. If a well-defended pedophile gains access to the group, he may be all too quick to recite typical incestuous conflicts and to take advantage of the optimistic prognosis afforded to incest offenders. His long-practiced skills of ingratiation and reassurance will propel him into figurehead status as the leader and a perfect example of the kind of total recovery and trust the program has afforded. Unfortunately, public testimonials ring sour, and the integrity of the program is threatened when the leader is found to be molesting children or using groups to expound his views on child love and consent.

The possible idiosyncracies and excesses of self-help zealots should not deter program planners from initiating and supporting affiliated self-help programs. Most medical programs have little precedent for active interaction with self-help groups; so the initial steps may appear intimidating. Professional responsibility, licensure, quality of care, liability, confidentiality, record keeping, fees for services, and a host of other professional considerations seem to exclude self-help involvement. Yet the experience can pay unexpected dividends if the reluctance and red tape can be overcome.

The Family Support Program at the Neuropsychiatric Institute, UCLA Center for the Health Sciences, is a good example of triumph over tradition. The program is a specialty child sexual abuse treatment project within the Psychiatric Clinic for Children, with full professional services as well as an active chapter of Parents United. The considerable difficulties of adapting university procedures to accommodate a self-help adjunct have faded in the light of the increased effectiveness, client enthusiasm, and community impact the Parents United component has contributed.

Rage

Victims of sexual abuse and their adult counterparts are not just ordinary people, any more than they are morally defective or constitutionally inferior. Whatever diverse factors have combined to allow for the reality of sexual abuse, there is a continuing legacy of hurt and anger. As long as the anger is turned inward and contained as self-hate, there may be little outward indication of danger to others. When the child grows up, the anger may explode against the child or children in the next generation, as already described in the section on peer-group contact. If the victim is a male, he is more likely than the female to grow up expressing his anger through violence and criminal behavior, as well as in relatively nonviolent molestation of children. Both women and men who are not ordinarily violent may be subject to dissociative states of homicidal frenzy or of carefully premeditated assassination and mass murder. The multiple personalities and the encapsulated rage states that characterize normal accommodation to sexual abuse are a poorly recognized source of substantial human suffering. Suffering spills from the reservoir of silent victims to their noncomplaining abused children and into the isolated, apparently wanton outbursts of violence against strangers.

Whatever their capacity for outward violence, the unhealed victims of abuse feel threatened by a poorly harnessed core of destructive energy. They may be passive and nonassertive for the very fear that any expression of negative feelings will erupt into a chain reaction of cosmic intensity. They tend to conceptualize themselves as a fragile layer of skin containing an expansive nucleus of indescribable badness that would contaminate and destroy anything it touched. The victim will call that core shit, scum, slime, or vomit, expressing obvious linkages to pregenital concepts of dirtiness, defiance, and badness. Sometimes there are direct associations to oral incorporation of semen or to anal penetration. Whatever the symbolic origins of the introject, it is endowed with demonic power in direct proportion to the outrageousness of the original assaults and in inverse proportion to the quality of maternal care and intervention experienced by the child. Because the introjected core is seen as so potentially destructive and because it is so charged with secrecy and self-blame, the victim has no permission for any reasonable discovery or outlet of the badness. Anything that scratches the surface is regarded as a threat, and any attempt to vent any of the pressure carries the imagined risk of dyscontrol and catastrophic explosion. As Shengold (1979, p. 555) writes:

> The most difficult task for the analyst is dealing with the patient's transference and projection. These are people whose bad expectations are of almost delusional intensity and whose rage is at a cannibalistic pitch (threatening destruction of both self- and parent imagoes as the rage begins to be felt). Fear of his rage is the greatest burden for the patient. It takes skill and empathy to help the patient in his struggle to tolerate the terrible anger, and in some cases it turns out to be too much for him to bear. And if this continues to be so, the responsible knowledge that the rage is there (*even* if it cannot be felt fully) enables the patient to think about it and to use it as a warning signal; this can make emotional growth possible.

The rage must be appreciated and respected by the therapist as well as the patient. Provocative challenges and unsupported probings for what may prove to be self-destructive or homicidal memories have no place in responsible treatment. Yet, when the rage comes up it should not be left unrecognized nor hastily covered in fear. Direct exercises in the constructive use of anger are often helpful. Role playing and even hypnotically abreactive excursions into the actual basis for the rage and the original pressure for self-scapegoating and helplessness can be therapeutic *if conducted within an environment of responsible care and support.* The therapist and the supportive peer group can assume a reparenting role to give adult endorsement and a kind of secondary mirroring to the experiences that seemed so totally reprehensible and devastating when seen through the eyes of the child in the absence of a redeeming primary parent. (Throughout this discussion I have mixed terms and concepts drawn from several theoretical perspectives and applied them to apparently incongruous levels of development. Since the sexual trauma occurs most often in latency years with a paternal figure, the emphasis on primary identity, basic trust, individuation, and other preoedipal, maternal issues may appear paradoxical. I can only assume that the betrayal of the paternal relationship and the consequent alienation and abandonment of any hope for maternal acceptance leave the child faced with a sense of annihilation that is comparable to the hungers and fears of early infant individuation and separation. There seems to be at least a fragmented or part-regression to primitive issues of survival.)

When rage is recognized, defined, and experientially rechanneled from the self and the concept of the bad child to a controlled focus on actually traumatic circumstances and actually hurtful caretakers, the patient experiences not explosion and punitive annihilation, but an unaccustomed sense of release and a capacity for self-control. Associated symptoms of somatic pain, neurasthenia, depression, and dissociative states tend to resolve with the reassignment of responsibility and anger. Conflicting personalities can be reconciled; hallucinations, childlike fantasy states, and ideas of reference can disappear. Grandiosity, paranoia, magical thinking, and self-mutilating punishment can mature into realistic self-acceptance and autonomy—all with the careful resolution of abusive conflicts within an atmosphere of responsible reparenting.

Such claims may in themselves sound grandiose and fantastic. It should be remembered that while victims of abusive atrocities may have spectacular conflicts and graphic symptoms, they are in fact *survivors* who have learned to protect themselves and to adapt to unbearable hazards. Their spectacular powers for recovery should be no less surprising than their remarkable feats of survival (Reagor, 1980).

Techniques of reparenting and optimal environments for support are still experimental, controversial, and anything but consistent, ranging from hospital programs to weekend marathons. The potentials and the limits for the most severely damaged survivors are not fully explored. There is a growing recognition that the large middle group of moderately symptomatic survivors, including most sexually abusive parents, can make remarkable readjustments and can achieve substantial recovery within programs incorporating traditional treatment skills combined with new appreciation of child-abusive dynamics and peer-group support.

Touch

There has been an empirical observation among workers in child abuse programs that adult clients turn to one another and to the staff for hugging as they resolve the conflicts of their own childhood and as they seek reassurance and permission as adults to confront their own fears and discomforts. Staff members have also learned that embraces can be an appropriate celebration of progress and a refreshing expression of endorsement and caring. Programs that develop comfort in physical contact and affectionate reinforcement seem to achieve better results, with less attrition of clients and staff, than programs that maintain more traditional distance and "adult" communication.

Child-damaged and child-damaging clients need something more meaningful than "adult" communication if they are going to learn to find trust in human contact. The vocabulary of reparenting, like any parenting, includes the nonverbal language of touch.

The child who has enough noncontingent caring and unrestricted holding in the first few years of life learns to spend increasing periods of time apart from physical contact as long as there remains full confidence that holding is never far away. With increasing sensory and cognitive development, the child learns to respond to smiles, words, material rewards, and complex behavioral conditioning for approval, in addition to a continuing pleasure in being held. Somewhere around school age for boys and only a few years later for girls, we begin to teach children that holding is for babies and that "growing up" requires taking pride in stoicism and self-reliance. Being held—like crying, thumb sucking, fuzzy blankets, and teddy bears—is put away as an unacceptable residue of childhood. After a certain age, we can be held only in the midst of pain, excitement, or, eventually, sexual arousal.

What is forgotten in this progression from closeness to distance, somatosensory to special senses, and concrete to abstract is that skin contact, warmth, and enfoldment constitute the *basic* human communication and the prototypic model for acceptance, affection, and reassurance. It is not so much that holding is "babyish" as that adult society tends to be "adultish"; that is, we become progressively alienated, defensive, and distrustful of dependency, intimacy, tenderness, and affectionate expression as we communicate with increasing numbers of abstractly related individuals. Rather than preserving and celebrating our small nucleus of touchworthy intimates, we seem to identify with the more alien society and to rely on abstract communication even within our most intimate and cherished circle of friends.

Some anthropologists and many students of family behavior believe that older children and adults develop a "skin hunger" that leaves individuals feeling vaguely unappreciated and unfulfilled and that can lead to reactive touching such as tickling, wrestling, tussling, and fighting, as well as premature and promiscuous sexual activity.

Sidney Simon (1976) writes about this hunger for human contact, as well as of the therapeutic benefits of compassionate contact. He defines the benefits of holding as "the simple but potent combination of touch itself and the human affirmation it delivers in a direct, unmistakeable, nonverbal way. . . . Beyond all this, it establishes in the very young the building material for better communication in all human relationships. . . . It results in people who are more open to the experience of life itself—people who feel secure enough to ask for what they want and need and who are generous enough to give others what they want in return" (Simon, 1976, p. 101).

Simon cites the primate research of Dian Fassey and of Harry and Margaret Harlow, as well as the human development observations of Rene Spitz, to illustrate what should be obvious to any observant human being: physical contact is indispensable for social development and emotional survival.

While Simon's prescription that every individual should have no less than three family hugs a day may seem humorous, I have no question that people who were abused as children and those who handle children abusively need permission and opportunity for noncontingent holding. For them, touching has become as often painful and possessive as protective, and caring has been dispensed only as a reward for performance or as a respite after an exhausting cycle of abuse. The sexually abused child has a special confusion about the meaning of touch, most often concluding that she or he is not worthy of touching apart from the painful ambivalence of being possessed by a parent.

For the patient deprived of basic trust and filled with self-hate and destructive rage, no real contact is possible short of an outstretched hand or an embrace. Smiles, words, and reassurances will not offset the individual's expectation of rejection and punishment. And physical distance in the face of verbal reassurances only affirms the conviction that the patient is in fact untouchable—too filthy, ugly, and dangerous to touch.

On the other hand, the therapist's capacity to feel and express genuine affection (token gestures are worse than nothing) through a solid hug can be redeeming and uniquely nourishing. As a patient wrote to her therapist in an incest-survivors' group:

Your hugs are warm: When you hold me I feel warm and good; most importantly warm.

Your hugs are caring: They prove a person is cared for. Who can willingly hold someone they dislike or hate?

Your hugs are respectful: They start and stop on time, allowing respect for someone's choice. When you hold me I feel I have the right to say what happens to my body. Not duty bound or forced. I can say *No*.

Your hugs are deeply satisfying: When you hold me the pain in my chest stops and the longing is fed. They last long enough to fill the whole of your goodness.

Your hugs are full: Arms surrounding completely and just tight enough to keep the goodness in and keep it from escaping. Close enough to really feel cared for.

Your hugs are encouraging: They make me feel that the dirt doesn't show. Who could put their arms around a mass of green slime? If it doesn't show and can't be felt perhaps there is a slight doubt that it exists.

Your hugs are everything a hug should be.

Thank you for your *hugs*.

For the child damaged during those years when touching was the only really meaningful contact, we cannot offer only abstract, adult-loaded, verbal signals of acceptance and approval. If the only therapeutic support available comes from someone who must maintain a formal separation and an objective distance from the patient, it is better that the realities of incestuous touching be left buried and unexplored.

The office practitioner in individual therapy is not in a comfortable setting to provide holding, especially with adult patients of the opposite sex or wherever there is a risk of eroticized or regressive transference. Group settings are likely to be more comforting to both patient and therapist, but the psychotherapist may still prefer to maintain a more traditional and more objective distance. In any case where the therapist does not provide the vital endorsement of holding, it is all the more important to endorse affectionate contact within an ancillarly peer group. The therapist who expects the sexually abused child or adult patient to confine all therapeutic communication within an individual, abstract relationship and who would reprimand the patient for "acting out" or "diluting the transference" by seeking ancillary caring and endorsement is guilty of a form of child neglect only slightly less damaging than the original assaults.

CONCLUSIONS

Any subject as diverse and controversial as child sexual abuse can be surveyed only superficially in a single chapter. Rather than offering the recapitulation of any specific program model or giving limited directions for complicated techniques of therapy, I have tried to stress underlying principles and goals.

It should be understood emphatically that recognition and the capacity for belief are the primary requisites for any effective response. Physicians must challenge their personal adult denial and theoretical objections in order to accomplish genuine objectivity and the capacity for subjective advocacy.

Reception room and emergency room recognition can be enhanced by improved diagnostic skills and protocols, as outlined or referenced in this chapter. Effective intervention requires also the documentation of behavioral and physical evidence as well as the willingness to report suspected abuse and to enter actively into both juvenile and criminal court procedures.

Follow-up support and optimum resolution of potential emotional consequences of child sexual abuse require specialty services not ordinarily available within pediatric or psychiatric centers. A specialized, integrated program for victims and their families can be established within a medical setting if adjustments can be made for the necessary paraprofessional self-help and community interagency networks required.

If the development of a specialty program is not practical within existing clinical resources, it is all the more important to participate in community councils on child abuse to encourage and support development of a free-standing sexual abuse treatment center.

Service elements and treatment philosophies for such a center are described. These elements are presented as a preliminary guide for program design and as an invitation to understand and to support such unfamiliar elements as reparenting therapies, peer-group techniques, self-help programs and compassionate holding.

Although this volume is directed to pediatric practice, this chapter includes treatment strategies for parents and for adult survivors of childhood sexual abuse as well as for child victims. Consideration of adult services and the involvement with the intergenerational cycle of child abuse establishes a supportive context for the immediate intervention and treatment of the child victim.

Aside from the introductory remarks concerning male victims of chronic sexual offenders, there is little reference to the treatment needs of sexually abused boys. While many boys and their parents seem to respond well to the general sexual abuse treatment program described here, there is an obvious need for better case finding and additional clinical experience with male victims.

There is also a pressing need for better recognition and diagnostic separation of chronic pedophiles from the more treatable incest offenders. Until more sensitive clinical measures can be devised, psychiatrists and other physicians are ill-prepared to define for the public or for the courts any reliably predictive guidelines for prognosis and potential treatment of sexual offenders against children.

While much remains to be learned, any physician participating in the recognition and reparenting of a sexually abused child should enjoy the opportunity to explore the last frontier of child abuse. The last frontier offers also a new threshold for understanding, treating, and preventing previously occult syndromes of disturbed behavior and mental illness.

REFERENCES

Armstrong, L. *Kiss Daddy Goodnight: A Speakout on Incest.* Hawthorn Books, New York (1978).

Benward, J., and Densen-Gerber, J. *Incest as a Causative Factor in Antisocial Behavior: An Exploratory Study.* Odyssey Institute, New York (1975).

Berliner, L., and Stevens, D. Special techniques for child witnesses. In *The Sexual Victimology of Youth,* L.G. Schultz, ed. Charles C. Thomas, Springfield (1979).

Berry, G.W. Therapeutic interventions with incestuous families. *Audio Digest, Psychiatry,* Vol. 6, No. 14 (July 25, 1977). (Recorded April 30, 1977, during presentation to the American Society for Adolescent Psychiatry, Toronto, Ontario.)

Bonaparte, M., Freud, A., and Kris, E., eds. *The Origins of Psychoanalysis, Letters To Wilhelm Fliess, Drafts and Notes: 1887-1902,* translated by E. Mosbacher and J. Strachey. Basic Books, New York (1954).

Breuer, J., and Frued, S. Studies on hysteria (1893-1895). In *The Complete Works of Sigmund Freud,* Vol. 2, J. Strachey, ed. Hogarth Press, London (1955).

Burgess, A.W., Holmstrom, L.L. Sexual trauma of children and adolescents: Pressure, sex and secrecy. *Nursing Clinics of North America, 10,* 551-563 (1975).

Burgess, A.W., Groth, A.N., Holmstrom, L.L., and Sgroi, S.M. *Sexual Assault of Children and Adolescents.* Lexington Books, Lexington, Mass. (1978).

Butler, S. *Conspiracy of Silence: The Trauma of Incest.* Bantam Books, New York (1979).

DeFrancis, V. *Protecting the Child Victim of Sex Crimes Committed by Adults.* American Humane Association, Denver (1969).

Ferenczi, S. (1933). Confusion of tongues between adults and the child. In *Final Contributions of the Problems and Methods of Psychoanalysis.* Basic Books, New York, (1955), pp. 155-167.

Finkelhor, D. *Sexually Victimized Children.* Free Press, New York (1979a).

———. What's wrong with sex between adults and children? Ethics and the problem of sexual abuse. *American Journal of Orthopsychiatry, 49,* 692-697 (1979b).

———. *Risk Factors in the Sexual Victimization of Children.* Family Violence Research Program, University of New Hampshire, Durham (1979c). (Publication pending)

Freud, S. (1896). The aetiology of hysteria. In *The Complete Works of Sigmund Freud,* Vol. 3, J. Strachey, ed. Hogarth Press, London (1955).

————. (1933). *The Complete Introductory Lectures of Psycho-Analysis*. W.W. Norton, New York (1966).

Gagnon, J.H. Female child victims of sex offenses. *Social Problems, 13,* 176–192 (1965).

Giaretto, H. Humanistic treatment of father-daughter incest. In *Child Abuse and Neglect: The Family and the Community,* R.E. Helfer and C.H. Kempe, eds. Ballinger, Cambridge, Mass. (1976).

————. Personal communication (1980).

Groth, A.N. Patterns of sexual assault against children and adolescents. In *Sexual Assault of Children and Adolescents,* A.W. Burgess, A.N. Groth, L.L. Holmstrom, and S.M. Sgroi, eds. Lexington Books, Lexington, Mass. (1978), pp. 3-24.

————. Personal communication (1980).

Jones, E. *The Life and Work of Sigmund Freud,* L. Trilling and S. Marcus, eds. Basic Books, New York (1961).

Landis, J. Experiences of 500 children with adult sexual deviants. *Psychiatric Quarterly Supplement, 30,* 91-109 (1956).

Martin, Lloyd. Personal communication (1980).

Myers, B.L. Incest: If you think the word is ugly, take a look at its effects. In *Readings in Sexual Abuse,* K. MacFarlane, ed. U.S. Government Printing Office (1981). (Publication pending)

National Committee for the Prevention of Child Abuse. *Dealing with Sexual Child Abuse,* Vol. 2, H. Donovan and R.J. Beran, eds. Chicago (1978).

Peters, J.J. Child rape: Defusing a psychological time bomb. *Hospital Physician, 9,* 46 (1973).

————. Children who are victims of sexual assault and the psychology of offenders. *American Journal of Psychotherapy, 30,* 398-412 (1976).

Queen's Bench Foundation. *Sexual Abuse of Children.* Project on Child Victims of Sexual Assault, San Francisco (1976).

Reagor, Pamela. Personal communication (1980).

Rush, F. The Freudian cover-up. *Chrysalis. 1,* 31-45 (1977).

Sgroi, S.M. Sexual molestation of children: The last frontier in child abuse. *Children Today, 4,* 18-21, 44 (1975).

————. Introduction: A national needs assessment for protecting child victims of sexual assault. In *Sexual Assault of Children and Adolescents,* A.W. Burgess, A.N. Groth, L.L. Holmstrom, and S.M. Sgroi, eds. Lexington Books, Lexington, Mass. (1978), pp. xv–xxii.

Shengold, L.L. Child abuse and deprivation: Soul murder. *Journal of the American Psychoanalytic Association, 27,* 533-599 (1979).

Simon, S. *Caring, Feeling, Touching.* Argus Communications, Niles, Ill. (1976).

Stoller, R.J. Hostility and mystery in perversion. *International Journal of Psycho-Analysis, 55,* 425-434 (1974).

Summit, R. Sexual child abuse, the psychotherapist, and the team concept. In *Dealing with Sexual Child Abuse,* Vol. 2, H. Donovan and R.J. Beran, eds. National Committee for the Prevention of Child Abuse, Chicago (1978), pp. 19-33.

Summit, R.C., and Kryso, J. Sexual abuse of children: A clinical spectrum. *American Journal of Orthopsychiatry, 48,* 237-250 (1978).

Weiss, J., Rogers, E., Darwin, M.R., and Dutton, C.F. A study of girl sex victims. *Psychiatric Quarterly, 29,* 1-27 (1955).

FILMS

Child Abuse: A Chain to be Broken. FMS Productions, Inc., Los Angeles, Calif.
Double Jeopardy. Motorola Teleprograms, Inc. Shiller Parks, Ill.

Appendix

Harborview Medical Center – Sexual Assault Center
Emergency Room Protocol – Child/Adolescent Patients

INFORMATION FOR ALL INVOLVED WITH PATIENT:

1. See immediately. Even though no physical trauma may be present, victims of sexual assault should receive high priority (immediately following acutely ill or injured patients).
2. Provide maximum support to parents as well as to the child/adolescent victim. Do not be judgmental nor allow emotional responses (e.g. anger, outrage) to interfere with providing optimal care.
3. Only those DIRECTLY involved in care should talk with the patient; give the patient and parents your name and explain your role.
4. Do not discuss sexual assault cases with anyone without the consent of the parent or legal guardian and the patient, if an adolescent.
5. "Rape" and "Sexual Assault" are legal, not medical terms. Do not use other than as "History of Sexual Assault".
6. The chart may be legal evidence. "Hearsay" statements from those who first see the child/adolescent may be admissible in court. All statements should be accurate, objective and legible.

EMERGENCY ROOM PERSONNEL:

1. Provide private facilities for the victim (ER 9 or the Quiet Room). Complete registration there.
2. Contact the ER physician immediately if there is evidence of moderate to severe physical trauma.
3. Obtain consent for care from the parents or legal guardian. If such consent cannot be obtained, contact the hospital administrator or the Juvenile Court for temporary consent. Examination of the adolescent should not be done without her/his consent unless a life-threatening emergency exists.
4. Contact social worker immediately.
5. If the assault occurred within the past 48 hours, contact the pediatric resident immediately. If the assault occurred more than 48 hours ago, the social worker will ascertain need for medical care.
6. The sexual assault tray and vaginal kit (containing Pedersen and pediatric specula) should be placed in exam room. (Check and replace items daily.)
7. Chaperone pelvic examination. A female chaperone (hospital employee) should be present for all pelvic examinations. Do not have the patient undress until just before the physical examination.

SOCIAL WORKER:

1. Assess immediate emotional needs of child and parents. Respond appropriately.
2. Confirm that the pediatric resident has been notified.
3. History: Obtain alone or in conjunction with the physician.
   a) Ascertain as much of the history as possible from parents or accompanying persons first, away from patient.
   b) See patient alone to obtain history (unless parent or other person is needed for support, i.e., in the very young child).
   c) Determine and use the patient's terminology for parts of the body, sexual acts, etc. Use aids, i.e., toys and picture books, as needed. Questions should be appropriate for age and developmental level.
   d) Obtain a directed history of the assault. Do not ask "why" questions, e.g., "Why did you go to his house?". Phrase questions in terms of "who, what, where, when", e.g., "Did the offender use oral, finger, penile contact to mouth, vulva, vagina, rectum?"; "How long ago did it happen?"; "Did penetration or ejaculation occur?"; "What kind of force, threat or enticement was used?"; "From whom did the patient seek help?".
   e) When the physician arrives, present history and impressions (out of patient's hearing) and complete history-taking conjointly.
4. Explain to patient and parents the reasons for questions asked, types of medical/legal tests needed, and possible treatment.
5. Obtain special consents, i.e., for photographs, release of clothing, release of information (specify to whom).
6. Assist with the physical examination, if indicated.
7. Discuss reporting to police and/or Children's Protective Service. Police may be contacted to come to the Emergency Room for an initial report.
8. Assessment and Counseling:
   a) Assess behavior and affect. Ascertain support systems of patient and family. Do not return child home unless the environment is safe. Document changes in housing.
   b) Explain anticipated emotional problems. Give patient and parents SAC handout.
   c) Encourage consulting with the Sexual Assault Center.
9. Record on Sexual Assault Report form services offered to patient:
   a) Medical appointment for follow-up care.
   b) Ongoing counseling or advocacy by SAC.
   c) Children's Protective Service referral, when indicated. (Referral to CPS is legally mandated when the offender is a family member or when the home environment does not protect the child from further sexual abuse.)
   d) Referrals made to other agencies.
   e) Victim's Compensation brochure, form, and brief explanation.

PHYSICIAN:

1. Medical History: Ascertain history from social worker and parents. Corroborate with patient. Do not needlessly repeat questions. Use "History of Sexual Assault" form #0245.

   a) Use vocabulary appropriate for age and developmental level. Use patient's words to describe and explain meaning if needed, i.e., "He put his 'thing' in me." (penis). Use picture books or toys as aids as needed.

   b) Ascertain activity post-assault: changes of clothing; bathing; douching; urinating; defecating; drinking.

   c) Obtain menstrual, contraceptive, VD history as needed.

   d) Obtain pertinent medical history: chronic illnesses; allergies; etc.

   e) Discuss VD prophylaxis, hormonal pregnancy prevention and abortion. Ascertain patient's feelings in these areas.

2. Approach to Examination:

   a) Be gentle and empathetic. Explain what you are doing in a calm manner and voice. Take time to relax the apprehensive patient.

   b) If supportive, have parent stay with child during the examination. Allow the adolescent the option of having whom s/he wishes to be present.

   c) Allow the patient to feel as much in control of his/her body during the exam as possible. Verbalize an understanding of his/her anxiety.

   d) Use appropriate gowns and drapes to ensure modesty and decrease feelings of vulnerability.

   e) Unless there is physical trauma which is apparent or must be ruled out, the complete examination does not need to be done (i.e. use of stirrups, speculum). All tests can be done with a glass pipette and cotton swabs.

      1) A small child may lie across the mother's lap in a "frog-leg" position.

      2) An older child may lie on the exam table in the same position.

      3) An adolescent may lie on the table in the same position or in stirrups.

   f) Use a REASONABLE approach. Use only those parts of the protocol appropriate for age of child and type of assault.

3. Physical Examination: Perform with hospital employee as chaperone.

   a) General: Document emotional status; general appearance of patient and clothing.

   b) Document areas of trauma on TRAUMAGRAM and describe in detail.

   c) Examine areas involved in sexual assault, i.e., oral, vaginal, rectal, penile. Very carefully document even minor trauma to these areas. Photograph areas of trauma as indicated (per evidence collection checklist).

   d) Ask patient to point with finger to exact area involved. Ask how much further offender penetrated.

   e) Describe developmental level (Tanner Stage), external genitalia, type and condition of hymen and diameter of introitus.

   f) Do exam as indicated by age of patient, type of assault and degree of injury. If injuries are extensive or cannot be determined due to lack of cooperation, consider examination and treatment under general anesthesia.

PHYSICIAN (continued):

4. Medical Tests:
   a) Culture body orifices involved for gonorrhea. If history is uncertain, culture all orifices.
   b) Obtain gravindex to rule out pregnancy as indicated.
   c) Obtain VDRL baseline. May be deferred in the young child or apprehensive adolescent.
5. Legal Tests:
   a) UV light — semen fluoresces. Examine areas of body and clothing involved (in dark after visual adaptation).
      1) Save clothing fluroescing for police (as per evidence collection checklist).
      2) Swab body areas fluorescing with saline moistened swabs. Place swabs in red top tubes. (Follow evidence collection checklist.)
   b) Wet mount preparation:
      1) Aspirate or swab areas of body involved (pharynx, rectum, vaginal pool). Saline moistened swabs may be used; however, aspiration with a glass pipette after flushing area with 2cc. of saline is preferred.
      2) Place drop of secretions on glass slide, plus drop of saline; examine immediately.
      3) Physician should examine several fields under high power with light source turned down. Document presence or absence of sperm and number of motile/nonmotile seen per high power field.
   c) Permanent smears:
      1) Physician will make two preparations. One slide will be a routine PAP from the endocervix and vaginal wall areas (may be deferred in child). The second slide will be a smear from the posterior vaginal pool, rectum, pharnyx as indicated. Obtain in the same manner as the Wet Mount.
      2) Put both slides promptly into the PAP bottle, back to back. DO NOT ALLOW TO AIR DRY. (Follow evidence collection checklist.)
      3) Physician will complete and sign PAP form noting "History of Sexual Assault; please do routine PAP and document presence or absence of sperm".
   d) Acid Phosphatase:
      1) Collect in same manner as for wet mount preparation.
      2) Place saline moistened swabs or secretions from pipette in red top tube. (Follow evidence collection checklist.)
   e) Other tests — as indicated or as police request (mainly to identify assailant, i.e., ABO antigens (collect as for acid phosphatase); fingernail scrapings; pubic hair combings.
6. Treatment:
   a) Injuries — treat and/or consult with other specialties as indicated. Give tetanus prophylaxis as indicated by history; follow CDC-Public Health recommendations (available in ER).

PHYSICIAN (continued):

 b) Pregnancy prophylaxis — may be given IF a vaginal assault occurred at mid-cycle, without contraception, and patient understands risks and side effects of estrogens to be given and is willing to have an abortion should pregnancy occur despite medication. *Do not prescribe* if there has been other unprotected intercourse during this cycle or any possibility of pre-existing pregnancy. Obtain a negative gravindex before instituting therapy.

   1) Hormonal therapy — Estinyl: 2.5 mg b.i.d. for 5 days. (Prepacks in ER).
   2) Antinauseant therapy — Bendectin (ii h.s. as needed for nausea and vomiting). Give routinely to use as needed. (Prepacks in ER).

 c) VD prophylaxis
   1) Not given routinely but as indicated, e.g., high patient anxiety, possibility patient will not return for follow-up care, known disease, multiple rapists.
   2) Therapy (over 12 years of age):
      a) Probenecid 1 gm orally + Ampillicin 3.5 gm orally stat; OR
      b) Probenecid 1 gm orally followed in 30 minutes by procaine penicillin G 4.8 million units IM; OR
      c) If penicillin allergy, spectinomycin 4 gm IM OR tetracycline 500 mgm q.i.d. x 4 days.
   3) Therapy (under 12 years of age): use age and weight appropriate dosages.

 d) Treatment for anxiety and/or difficulty sleeping — as indicated (rarely needed in children under 12 years; use age appropriate dosage when given). Adult therapy as follows:
   1) Mellaril 10 mgm one-half hour before sleep (may repeat once, if necessary; do not exceed 20 mgm/day. Give a 3-day supply (60 mgm); OR
   2) Valium 5 mgm one-half hour before sleep (may repeat once p.r.n.). Do not exceed 10 mgm/day. Give 3-day supply (30 mgm).

7. Final Care
 a) Verbally express concern and availability for help as needed.
 b) Reinforce social worker information; reinforce that patient is physically intact and is not responsible for the assault/abuse.
 c) Discuss medical problems which may arise and encourage family to call as needed.

8. Final Diagnosis
 a) History of Sexual Assault.
 b) Presence or absence of sperm.
 c) Specific diagnosis of injuries, contusions, lacerations, etc.
 d) Other pertinent medical diagnoses.

PHYSICIAN (continued):

9. Follow-up
    a) Pediatric Clinic appointment in one week.
    b) Repeat gonorrhea cultures at follow-up visit; VDRL in 8 weeks; other as indicated.
    c) Consultation from other specialties as indicated.

7/78
Sexual Assault Center
Harborview Medical Center
325 Ninth Avenue
Seattle, WA   98104

11

The Psychological Effects of Genetic Disorders in Children and Their Parents

Isabelle Leddet-Chevallier and Steve Funderburk

It is nearly impossible to make statements about the personal significance of being marked genetically deviant. The most immediate significance of such knowledge for a person revolves about its impact on his concept of himself as a complete person and the interpersonal and social impact on his self-concept. These psychological effects of genetic disease impact on the affected child, his parents, and, indeed, on the entire family.

To be affected by, or to be a carrier of, a genetic disorder may not mean illness or disability in the common sense. Health, however, can be thought of in terms of physical, psychological, and social adequacy. "For most people, in fact, health does not mean so much the absence of disease as the ability to conduct life according to personal choices and social conventions" (Dubos, 1977). Accordingly, the significance of carrier status resides more in what it means for the individual in terms of his psychological and social functioning. The carrier individual may perceive that he has a severe personal problem if he interprets his genetic endowment as a punishment for his own conduct. The genetic disorder may have significance for personal plans of work and his concept of his personal integrity. A diminished self-esteem can be inadvertently exacerbated by counselors who employ imagery that is loaded for the counselee. For example, to speak about hemoglobinopathies as "conditions of the blood" can parallel the "bad blood" imagery many people use for undesirable hereditary traits (Headings, 1979). Furthermore, if a person discovers that he possesses or transmits a defective gene, his self-image is affected, and he often experiences feelings of shame. He may think he is being punished for something he has done in the past. "While our understanding of genetics has shifted from the realm of animism to naturalism, and the change in our view of genetics from social problems to medical issues has greatly reduced the chance that individuals will interpret carrier status as a sign of personal worth, this remains something of a problem" (Sorenson, 1974).

In a number of cities, screening programs for hemoglobin disorders (e.g., sickle-cell anemia, beta-thalassemia) or metabolic diseases (e.g., Tay-Sachs disease) are identifying large numbers of healthy individuals as carriers of a single mutant gene. The commonly stated goal of such screening and subsequent counseling is the prevention of the birth of an affected child. Current efforts to educate, test, and counsel may, however, cause anxiety and generate guilt, resentment, and frustration or inhibit the development of personal self-esteem and racial pride. The public image of "defectiveness" in the individual's biology, necessitating publicly financed prevention programs, may convince the individual with a genetic trait or disease that society is opposed to these groups of individuals marked with less adequate ancestry than other populations (Headings, 1979).

Discovery of a genetic disorder often creates the initial reactions of shock, disbelief, anger, and depression. Once the mourning period is over, the next stop concerns decision making. Presented with the risk of their situation, individuals with a genetic trait or disease have to decide whether to consider this risk in the selection of a marital partner or in having children if they marry or are married to a person with the same trait. The presence of fear, anxiety, and apprehension sometimes creates an emotional climate that compromises their ability to make decisions in their best interest.

Repercussions of a genetic disorder are probably most immediate and most likely to alter life expectations and experiences for prospective parents. Probably for the great majority of individuals, the ability to have children is self-fulfilling. Accordingly, the presence of a genetic trait or disease in adolescents and potential parents affects significantly their images of sexual and parenting competence. Furthermore, when a recurrence risk is linked with reproduction, future parents may conclude erroneously that sexual or reproductive incompetence is implied.

Individual perceptions of risk differ widely. Some patients interpret a 10 percent risk as high; others interpret this risk as low. In some cases of dominant single-gene disease, parents consider a risk of 50 percent acceptbale. These differences are in the reaction to the perceived risk: 10 percent is seen as the same level of risk by all, but some feel they can handle the consequences of taking this chance, while others feel they cannot.

> The patient, K.S., presented at 28 years of age for further surgical repair of cleft lip, palate, and lip pits. She had a family history consistent with autosomal dominant inheritance. She was attractive, sociable, married, and successfully employed as an elementary school teacher. She and her husband sought genetic counseling to confirm their impression that her condition was inherited. When informed of the 50 percent recurrence risk for each of their future children, K.S. said that she did not wish to have

children unless she could be assured that they would not have externally visible facial clefting. Both she and her husband stated that they would want to abort an affected fetus if prenatal diagnosis of facial clefting were possible. K.S. reasoned that although she had made a reasonable adjustment, she would not want a child to go through her early experiences of repeated hospitalizations, speech therapy, and mild facial disfigurement. In contrast to most medical professionals, who view cleft lip and palate as remedial and therefore a relatively benign malformation, K.S. had a more severe sense of the burden of her disorder.

As pointed out by Leonard, Chase, and Childs (1972), it may be the sense of burden imparted by the disease, rather than the magnitude of the recurrence risk, that primarily affects reproductive attitudes. It appears that socially acceptable justifications for (or against) childbearing are as important as personally relevant issues in the actual deliberation. Informed with facts, parents frequently make decisions that least disturb their sense of personal or family equilibrium, whether or not prevention of the disease is accomplished by the decision (Headings, 1979).

A new sense of responsibility in future parents has been provided by the availability of prenatal diagnosis. This diagnostic procedure, combined with abortion when a defect is diagnosed, permits the family to participate actively in determining some aspects of the biological quality of its progeny. On the other hand, a misunderstanding of these new techniques may lead to an idealized conception of perfection in the offspring, prompted by the common tendency to see one's children not as independent beings, but as extensions of oneself. Production of a defective child is in that sense a reflection upon the parent. It should be clear that amniocentesis involves more than a simple, ordinary medical procedure. Major psychosocial concomitants involved may have important long-term consequences for the couple and their family.

One of the most difficult problems faced by the counselor involves helping couples at risk to resolve differences of opinion or conflicts in decision making. Some physicians and counselors may imply that couples at risk should not have children. This can exaggerate deep-seated guilt reactions in persons who by accident or design later have a child with the disease. They could be burdened with undue guilt for not having followed the implied advice. Individuals with a genetic trait should be presented with factual information necessary to have a balanced picture of the disease, rather than with the counselor's judgment or opinion as to recommendations. The genetic counselor should be a "helper" and not a "director" as far as the family is concerned (Weiss, 1976). Recommending to couples with the potential for having children with a genetic disease that they should not reproduce could unduly influence them to comply, thereby denying themselves the sense of fulfillment achieved through procreation.

Some parents are strongly determined to procreate, whatever the risk of having a genetically affected child. This may result from their focusing on the possibility of having a normal child, diffusing responsibility, or recognizing that they had already coped with the worst. This mechanism of thought allows them to perceive their situation as manageable and facilitates their decision to try.

In other cases involving a difficult procreative decision, inefficient contraceptive practices may be found. Common to parents who have not made firm reproductive choices is the lack of a clear perception that they can cope with the worst. In this way, a "nondecision" can be seen as a valid alternative to a deliberate choice of reproduction or contraception: it is a choice not to decide, a choice of "fatalism" made when one does not want to exert control (Lippman-Hand and Fraser, 1979). When prenatal diagnosis is available, it may be a powerful neutralizer, which provides a socially accepted way of avoiding having an affected child while still maintaining the ability to become a parent.

THE CHILD

Concomitantly with the physical disability of many hereditary diseases, children also inherit psychosocial problems. One of the most important aspects is that genetic conditions are often irreversible: "One characteristic is the permanency of the genetic diagnosis. Once made, the genetic diagnosis ipso facto defines an irreversible condition" (Schild, 1979). Thus, crucial life tasks and aspirations may be affected by the genetic disorder.

Chronic Illness

For many children with genetic disorders (i.e., cystic fibrosis or muscular dystrophy), there are multiple lifelong medical, emotional, social, and financial difficulties that restrict everyday existence. Such problems as repeated treatments, hospitalizations, and experiences of pain are inherent in chronic illness. Depression may be experienced by the child very early in life when he is separated from his familial milieu, particularly when he is hospitalized. Spitz (1945) described hospitalization as an etiologic factor in psychiatric conditions in early childhood. Varying degrees of depression may be experienced by hospitalized children, with feelings of helplessness and fear of abandonment (i.e., fear that they will be left to experience the illness without appropriate help, intervention, or psychological support).

Feelings of helplessness may also result from exposure to painful procedures inherent in medical care. Often little effort is made to interpret the hospital world to the child, particularly to explain when painful procedures are going to occur; the hospitalized child can live in constant fear of the unknown. He may develop resentment at having the disease and toward his parents for passing on the disease to him. The illness and its manifestations need to be explained in terms understandable to the child. If he is not given clear, honest, simple explanations, he creates answers for himself, many of which are erroneous. The child may imagine a cause and effect relationship, because this is a child's natural mode of thinking. He may firmly believe that his illness and pain are forms of punishment for bad thoughts or past behavior.

There are many barriers to the development of a sense of mastery over disease that may diminish the child's sense of self-esteem. Children with sickle-cell anemia, for instance, are powerless to influence fatigue, or time of onset, frequency, duration, or intensity of the crisis. Some may become hypochondriacal and experience more pain and fatigue than can be accounted for by their physical condition. Adolescents may realize that the disease is incurable, resulting in reduced life span, and that death from the disease can occur at any age. Feelings of despair and preoccupations with death may be so strong as to affect crucial decisions such as career, marriage, and children.

A child with a chronic illness has intrinsic anxieties and faces social, educational, and vocational restrictions. Failure to deal with these psychosocial problems may result in a greater handicap to the patient than the disease itself. Because of repeated treatments and hospitalizations, a chronically ill child experiences slowing in his educational career, with interruptions of normal activities, physical limitations, and difficulties in attending school. Underachievement may threaten his sense of self-worth, and his ego development may be impaired.

Parents tend to be overprotective. This leads to frictions and intensifies family anxiety, generating behavior problems in the child. Parental overprotection may at times foster a closer family relationship, but it usually tends to inhibit normal exploratory activity in the child. It is essential to help the parents promote autonomy and independence in their disabled child.

Normal adolescent development is characterized by sexual maturation, psychological separation from the parents, and the need to be increasingly independent. An adolescent with a chronic illness may remain in a passive, dependent relationship with his parents. His view of life and of his own potential may be constricted, and gradual withdrawal from normal relationships may occur. He may not have the universal dreams and aspirations of adolescents, and his self-esteem may be inadequate.

Another normal developmental step in adolescence is the reformulation and consolidation of body image. Common strategies used to cope with chronic illness or physical disability include avoidance and overcompensation. "Denial appears to be the principal coping strategy used to deal with the impairment of the body construct as well as the issue of dependent" (Fischman, 1979).

This 13-year-old girl was referred for multiple cysts of the jaw. She had associated small, pedunculated nevi over the neck and shoulders and palmar pits. The diagnosis of autosomal dominant basal cell nevus syndrome was made. The recurrence risk to her future children was not understood, and she refused orthodontic care for her multiple cysts. In refusing this necessary treatment and in failing to comprehend the hereditary risks, she was acting as if the disease were not present.

Phenylketonuria (PKU)

Screening and treatment efforts are resulting in an ever increasing group of physically and intellectually normal PKU children.

Mental development in most PKU children appears to be inversely related to the age of onset of dietary treatment (Shear, Willman, and Nyhan, 1974). Children treated early show normal levels of intelligence, although some may show mild to moderate degrees of visual-perceptual difficulties (Schild, 1979).

Children with PKU are frequently reported to show behavioral abnormalities, communication defects, and extreme hyperactivity. Strict dietary treatment strongly affects the mother-child relationship, and the child is more likely to have behavioral problems that usually center around food. Parents of PKU children tend to be overprotective and to inhibit normal exploratory activities of their children. This may account for some of the learning difficulties observed in treated PKU children and for their reported deficits in verbal expression.

As these children grow up, other issues, such as diet discontinuation, academic performance, peer relationships, and secondary emotional aspects come more into focus and demand the attention of the caring professional. In particular, when adolescent girls with PKU approach the reproductive age and face the consequences of childbearing (gestational dietary restriction to prevent abnormal fetal development), they will have to be familiarized with the multiple problems of womanhood. Thus professionals must recognize their responsibility and obligation to discuss with parents and their PKU daughters the complexities of maternal PKU. In order to help PKU girls during adolescence in a constructive way, the emotional elements prevailing in adolescence, such as dependence, ambivalence, and secretiveness should be understood. It is also important to recognize the parents' normal reluctance and fear of discussing subjects of sex and reproduction with a teenager. This reluctance is amplified in parents of PKU daughters, since the parents carry the burden of knowing the genetic implications of PKU.

Congenital Anomalies

If a chronic genetic disease affects the child and his family in everyday life, the existence of congenital anomalies, especially facial disfigurements, also affects strangers and society itself. "The effects are reciprocal, since all of these provide feedback information and, in a sense, a social mirror in which reflections are interpreted by the anomalous person" (Clifford, 1973, p. 2). Physical anomalies and disfigurements have psychological effects on the child's feelings and personality development, which are reinforced by familial and societal reactions.

Very early in life, feeding difficulties because of oral clefts, for instance, or difficulties in holding the child and taking care of him may distort mother-child interaction. This very early relationship may condition future personality development and psychic life (Spitz, 1965), and a disruption in the relationship may lead to behavior problems and personality disturbances (Bowlby, 1969). Because the existence of a disability may interfere with the primary need for mothering, it is presumed that frustration is introduced into the relationship, the effects of which will be evidenced in later life.

Attention is focused on the face early in the life of the infant. Smiling behavior occurs by one month of age and is looked upon as an important milestone in the socialization process (Spitz, 1965). Emotional problems relating to disfigurement may be transmitted to the child by his parents and other members of society.

The congenitally disabled child, however, is not aware of any abnormality until he can appreciate differences between people and until his difference is called to his attention. According to Friedman (1978), patients start to realize that they are different from other children between the ages of two and three years. The disabled child then incorporates the values of the physically normal and adopts the cultural standards of attractiveness. Concomitantly, he experiences society's negative attitudes toward the disabled, and as he perceives how he is valued by others, his self-concept is affected. Disabled children make poor adjustments later in life not only because of their functional insufficiency, but also because of the psychic abnormalities fostered in them.

Handicapped persons have been socially labeled, imputing that they are different from other people and that the difference is undesirable. Labeling may engender a sense of shame, partly in response to the social stigma that may be attached to the label. Stigmatization, in turn, may lead to social rejection. Common reactions to disfiguring faults include ridicule, with use of sobriquets and accusations of wrongdoing.

Society considers the handicapped inferior not only physically, but in every other sense. Facial appearance influences our judgment of intelligence, and mental illness is often attributed to the disfigured. Handicapped children may appear to be mentally retarded, while actually being only socially retarded as a result of rejection and isolation. Handicapped children are exposed to fewer social experiences, as many parents tend to avoid social contacts because of the child's appearance. His striking appearance focuses a certain amount of attention on him, and the staring of normal persons is difficult to avoid. Hypersensitivity may develop in reaction to this, and the disabled child may make increased demands for personal attention.

Normal persons experience feelings of unease and ambivalence and tend to alter their behavior in the presence of a person with a visible disability. They are less spontaneous and distort their opinions in ways they feel would be more acceptable to the disabled (Richardson, 1976). These negative feelings represent a strong barrier to effective interpersonal relations; normal persons tend to avoid the disabled, who in turn experience difficulties in getting jobs, making friends, and getting married.

Possible reaction patterns to social distance and disability may range from withdrawal, to hostility with antisocial behavior, to successful coping with the situation. A comfortable acceptance of self eventually may be attained, perhaps because being physically disabled or restricted from normal activity allows more time for self-evaluation and self-knowledge (Goffman, 1968). A quest for normality is often seen in people with a genetic disease, as their lives are plagued with the exception. In this respect, denial is a universal reaction, a refusal to accept abnormality.

Despite physical disability and disease-related familial and social problems, many individuals with a genetic disease choose to marry and to have children. "A concern to prove one's manhood or womanhood, an adequacy of sexual performance, and an ability to freely choose one's activities, may appear to the individual to be placed in jeopardy by this (genetic) condition" (Headings, 1979).

In this young woman a diagnosis of bilateral retinoblastoma was made in early childhood and treatment ensued. Radiation-induced tumors progressively invaded one orbita and mouth cavity, resulting in surgical excision and a prosthesis in one eye and the mouth. The patient experienced the conditions of the blind and disfigured. She knew that her cosmetic appearance did not fit with societal standards, and because of her disabilities she experienced rejection, isolation, and difficulty in making friends. However, she became a pianist and succeeded in being good at her occupation. She fought to become independent, though she recognized her dependence on her mother. She learned to commute via public transportation. Presented with the fact of autosomal dominant inheritance with 50 percent recurrence risk for her future offspring, she expressed the hope of getting married and being able to have a normal child. Her mother, in contrast, thought that her daughter should not even consider having children, who might bear the same burden she had to bear. The patient coped with her genetic condition and sought normality through normal reproductive desires.

Progress in cosmetic surgery and prostheses can improve social acceptance and the physical abilities of disabled and disfigured children. Some parents, however, may seek surgery as a solution to all of the child's associated behavioral and developmental difficulties. It is essential that professionals be aware of such problems and attempt some form of psychological intervention prior to surgical correction.

THE PARENTS

The presence of a developmental problem in a child nearly always has some adverse psychological effect on the parents (Solnit and Stark, 1961), and the presence of a genetic or inherited component may add to this psychological burden. Olshansky (1962) emphasized that the parent of a mentally defective child suffers from chronic sorrow, and that this sorrow is a natural response to a tragic fact. In reviewing his earlier observations, Farber (1975) proposed that the family usually chooses a course of minimal adaptation in response to crises that recur in the process of caring for the mentally retarded child.

Controlled studies, however, have not always demonstrated such a devastating effect on the families of mentally retarded individuals. Davis and MacKay (1973) reported on a survey from Belfast of 70 families with a mentally subnormal child. Twenty-eight of the families were matched with a control group of families. In the matched groups, there was no difference in the incidence of separation or divorce, physical health of the parents, mental health as evidenced by hospital admissions or neurotic symptoms, personality disorders such as alcoholism, or employment. However, the matched families of disabled children had fewer social outings and fewer holidays. A study of the effect of infants with Down's syndrome on the family was reported by Gath (1977). Thirty families with a newborn infant with Down's syndrome were matched with 30 families with a normal baby. Both groups were followed for 18 to 24 months and were interviewed six times. Few differences could be found in the mental or physical health of the two groups of parents, but marital breakdown or severe marital disharmony was found in nine of the Down's syndrome families and in none of the controls.

In reporting results of interviews with parents of children with a variety of malformations, Irvin, Kennell, and Klaus (1976) stated that few studies have examined how parental reactions might vary according to the disabling condition in the child. The authors proposed that mental development, number of anomalies, heritability, and correctability—all may influence ultimate parental reactions and adaptations to the child's disorder. It seems reasonable to suppose that the severity and duration of the parents' initial reaction would be greatly influenced by the nature of the child's condition.

In an assessment of parents' mental and physical health, Blumenthal (1967) found a similar degree of illness among parents of children with mental retardation, cystic fibrosis, and PKU. The intent of this study was to look for any possible heterozygote effect among carrier parents of children with a recessive disorder affecting brain development (i.e., PKU). The finding of no difference among parents of children with mental retardation, cystic fibrosis, and PKU, in addition to showing no heterozygote effect, also suggests no secondary psychological effect on the family from the presence of mental retardation in the child. However, the severity and chronicity of pulmonary disease in cystic fibrosis, even though mental development is usually normal, make this a serious disabling condition in the child. Therefore, the parents' perception of burden of disease in children with mental retardation, cystic fibrosis, and PKU may be comparable.

It may be enlightening to review results of studies examining the psychosocial effects of physical defects that are usually limited and surgically correctable. A relatively rapid dissipation of the effects of the original shock was reported for parents of infants with cleft lip and palate (Clifford, 1968), and feelings of depression lasted only up to four days in parents of infants with cleft lip and palate (Koch-Schulte, 1968). Wirls and Plotkin (1971) compared the results of projective personality tests between 66 cleft palate only ($N = 32$) and lip and palate ($N = 34$) children between the ages of 7 and 14, and an equal number of siblings within the same age range. The author speculated that there may be many reasons why cleft lip and palate children might develop personality differences: special problems of care and feeding during infancy, traumas of surgery early in life, parental reactions, facial disfigurement, hearing loss, and defective speech. However, the number of significant differences between the patients and their siblings was fewer than expected by chance. In reviewing several of his studies of families of children with cleft lip and palate, Clifford (1973) concluded that families with handicapped children do not show more overprotectiveness than families with unaffected children and that the handicapped families do not show more disintegration than families with normal children. The author does not discuss the possibility that more chronically handicapping conditions, such as those with mental retardation or multiple malformations, might have a more adverse effect on the family.

One would also expect that the availability of specialized services and social agencies would influence parents' reactions to the birth of a child with a genetic disorder. Waisbren (1980) compared 30 families with handicapped children residing in California to 30 families in Denmark. Although support systems were generally more available in Denmark, the Danish families did not show any better adjustment than the California families. The author concluded that the psychological impact, rather than the practical aspects of the child's condition, had the most effect on the parents. Voysey (1972), in discussing the effects of a mentally retarded child on the parents, suggested that the parents' style of coping is not determined by the child's disability alone, that the parental inter-actional style remains to some extent a negotiable issue.

Even though the nature of the child's disability must certainly influence parental reactions, it is revealing that numerous authors report similar parental reactions to a diversity of handicapping conditions. The initial reactions of shock, denial, anger, guilt, sorrow, and depression are recurring themes from authors who have worked with handicapped families. Without giving specific data, Tisza and Gumpertz (1962) reported their findings from interviews with parents, especially mothers, and from observations in a well-care clinic, among babies who were born with cleft palate. The authors reported that mothers reacted with strong feelings of hurt, disappointment, and helpless resentment. They wanted to know the cause of the malformation and blamed medical procedures, previous diet, lack of vitamins, and relatives or medical professionals. Parental anxieties several months after the birth of the child related to irregular dentition and teething difficulty, excessive drooling, difficult chewing and swallowing, differences in amount and quality of vocalization, and fear of intellectual impairment or actual mental retardation.

Drotar et al. (1975) reported similar findings from interviews of parents with 20 children with a range of malformations. The interviews took place 7 days to 60 months after birth. These interviews demonstrated the parental reactions of shock, denial, sadness and anger, adaptation, and reorganization. Beal (1962) and Friedman (1978) reported very similar reactions among parents of children with congenital amputations. The latter stressed the concept that the impact of the handicapping condition is determined more by psychological and emotional reactions than by physical limitations. He reasoned that physical limitations can be largely overcome with prostheses, specialized training, and equipment, but that the patient's attitude toward his handicap may limit the effectiveness of rehabilitation.

Numerous authors have reported parental overprotection of their physically handicapped child and interpreted this to be a result of conscious or subconscious rejection, neglect, or death wish for the defective infant. Beal (1962, p. 146) gave an example of a mother who was extremely and pathologically overprotective of her child with multiple anomalies. Only years after the birth of the child was the mother able to state that after first seeing the child she sat in a room by herself and thought over and over, "Couldn't they get rid of it?" The author interpreted the mother's overprotectiveness as resulting from long-term guilt for feelings of rejection toward the child. Gurney (1958), in presenting

the results of findings based on interviews with parents of 25 children with congenital amputation, gave an example of a child who was severely emotionally
(but not cognitively) retarded due to the extreme degree of maternal guilt and
overprotection. That author felt that parents could be classified into three
groups with increasing severity of maladaptation. In the first group, the parents
had sufficiently coped with the traumatic experience of having given birth to a
child with an anomaly and had freed themselves from self-blame. Consequently,
they could discuss the disability realistically and openly, could communicate
understanding to the child, and be helpful to him. In the second group were
parents who were bewildered by the problems, who continued to have feelings
of self-blame, and who worried about reactions of strangers, friends, and relatives to the amputation or prosthesis. Parents in this group, however, had the
strength to look at their reactions and concerns. At least one parent of each
couple in the second group had the capacity to look at his reactions and make
use of help. The third group consisted of parents who attempted to absorb the
child in their own needs and conflicts or who isolated the child through avoidance of communication; who had withdrawn from close association with other
family members; and who in defense denied the need for help. The author concluded that these parents were extremely guilt-ridden and overprotective to the
extent that they could not deal realistically with the amputation and with
prostheses.

From his clinical experience with the limb-deficient child, Friedman (1978)
stated that parental rejection and physical abuse of the limb-deficient child
occurs, and even infanticide is not uncommon. He stated that mothers may
frequently, consciously or unconsciously, kill, abandon, or ignore the abnormal
child, and that compensation for these feelings results in overprotection. In addition, many amputees have a fear of genetic transmission of the disability, and
this exists even for traumatically acquired amputations. The author concluded
that long-term progress in minimizing the psychic consequences of disability will
require more societal acceptance of handicapping conditions.

The Group for the Advancement of Psychiatry (1963) applied the same
dynamic explanation for parental overprotection of the mentally retarded child.
They reasoned that the parent actually has guilt for rejection of or death wishes
toward the child, and that this guilt leads to irrational overprotection. Targum
and Weiss (1980, p. 23) stated that parental overinvolvement with the child may
be a defense against rage and anger at the child for having been born defective:
"The narcissistic pride which parents invest in their children may lead to severe
damage to the parents' sense of self. . . . The baby is often a composite of repre-
sentations of the self and love objects. . . . The parents are faced with the
unenviable task of accepting a defective child of their own creation." In the case
of a father of a Tay-Sachs infant, brief psychotherapy revealed a sense of
personal defectiveness, and for the first time in his life the father was forced to

confront his own feelings of inadequacy. These authors stressed that the genetic nature of a defect probably accentuates such parental reactions. It should be reiterated, however, that there has not been a systematic investigation to determine whether there is a correlation between the intensity and quality of parental reactions and the severity and nature of the child's handicapping condition.

Crisis Intervention

Numerous authors cited above (Beal, 1962; Tisza and Gumpertz, 1962; Paulson and Stone, 1973; Drotar et al., 1975; Waisbren, 1980) reached the common conclusion that some form of crisis intervention for parents of young handicapped infants would serve to maximize long-term parental adjustment. The work of Caplan (1961) provided a theoretical basis for the potential benefits of mental health intervention during times of crisis. It is possible that the eventual adaptation to an initial agonizing situation with severely wounded self-esteem could result in an emotionally strong individual. Goffman (1968) wrote about the "deep philosophy" in persons with stigma, and Voysey (1972) spoke of the more positive self-image in parents of handicapped children. Whether the type of therapeutic intervention during times of crisis should be tailored to the type of handicapping condition remains to be determined from future investigations.

At whatever stage of contact with the family, the professional needs to understand the dynamics of parental reactions. It is useful to view these as normal emotional reactions, and thereby to show respect and validation toward the parents and their feelings. As emphasized by Olshansky (1962), if the professional accepts chronic sorrow as a natural rather than a neurotic response, he can be more effective in helping the parent achieve the goal of increased comfort in living with and managing a mentally defective child. This advice can probably be generalized to many emotional reactions among parents of children with a variety of genetic disorders. Rather than suggesting to parents that their specific anxieties and concerns are not based on fact, it is probably more helpful to state that their feelings and reactions are normal. For example, accepting parents' feelings of guilt, rather than negating them, may leave the parents with some sense of power and control (Kessler, 1979). Clearly there are instances, however, when the professional needs to recognize the abnormal or maladjusted family reaction. The parent who has become overtly depressed over feelings of guilt and is burdened with the care of the affected child or the parent whose excessive overprotection is blocking the child's development clearly may benefit from mental health intervention. It is important to recognize such examples of pathological adaptation and to seek professional intervention for the family.

This research was supported in part by the UCLA Mental Retardation/Child Psychiatry Division and USPHS grants MCH-927, HD-04612, HD-05615, and HD-06576.

REFERENCES

Beal, L.L. The impact of an anomalous child on those concerned with his welfare. *Orthopedic and Prosthetic Application Journal, 16,* 144–147 (1962).

Blumenthal, M.D. Mental illness in parents of phenylketonuric children. *Journal of Psychiatric Research, 5,* 59–74 (1967).

Bowlby, J. *Attachment and Loss,* Vol. 1. Basic Books, New York (1969).

Caplan, G. *Prevention of Mental Disorders in Children; Initial Explorations.* Basic Books, New York (1961), p. 13.

Clifford, E. Effects of giving birth to a cleft lip-palate baby. Paper presented at the Plastic Surgery Research Council, Durham, N.C. (1968).

– – –. Psychosocial aspects of orofacial anomalies: Speculations in search of data. *Orofacial Anomalies: Clinical and Research Implications.* Proceedings of the American Speech and Hearing Association, Report No. 8 (1973), pp. 2–29.

Davis, M., and MacKay, D.N. Mentally subnormal children and their families. *Lancet, 2,* 974–975 (1973).

Drotar, D., Baskiewicz, A., Irwin, N., Kennell, J., and Klaus, M. The adaptation of parents to the birth of an infant with a congenital malformation: A hypothetical model. *Pediatrics, 56,* 710–717 (1975).

Dubos, R. The despairing optimist. *The American Scholar,* 424–430 (1977).

Farber, B. Family adapatations to severely mentally retarded children. In *The Mentally Retarded Child in Society: A Social Science Perspective,* M.J. Begab and S.A. Richardson, eds. University Park Press, Baltimore (1975), pp. 247–266.

Fischman, S.E. Psychological issues in the genetic counseling of cystic fibrosis. In *Genetic Counseling. Psychological Dimensions,* S. Kessler, ed. Academic Press, New York (1979), pp. 153–165.

Friedmann, L.W. The limb-deficient child. In *The Psychological Rehabilitation of the Amputee.* Charles C. Thomas, Springfield (1978), pp. 77–83.

Ibid

Gath, A. The impact of an abnormal child upon the parents. *British Journal of Psychiatry, 130,* 405–410 (1977).

Goffman, E. *Stigma: Notes on the Management of Spoiled Identity.* Penguin Books, London (1968).

Group for the Advancement of Psychiatry (GAP). *Mental Retardation: A Family Crisis—The Therapeutic Role of the Physician.* Formulated by the Committee on Mental Retardation, Report No. 56, New York (December, 1963).

Gurney, W. Parents of children with congenital amputation. *Children, 5,* 95–100 (1958).

Headings, V.E. Psychological issues in sickle cell counseling. In *Genetic Counseling. Psychological Dimensions*, S. Kessler, ed. Academic Press, New York (1979), pp. 153–165.

Irvin, N.A., Kennell, J.H., and Klaus, M.H. Caring for parents of an infant with a congenital malformation. In *Maternal-Infant Bonding*, M.H. Klaus and J.H. Kennell, eds. C.V. Mosby, St. Louis (1976), pp. 167–250.

Kessler, S., ed. *Genetic Counseling; Psychological Dimensions*. Academic Press, New York (1979).

Koch-Schulte, R. Family adjustment to the newborn with cleft lip and palate. Paper presented at the American Cleft Palate Association, Miami Beach, Fla. (1968).

Leonard, C.O., Chase, G.A., and Childs, B. Genetic counseling: A consumer's view. *New England Journal of Medicine, 287*, 433–439 (1972).

Lippman-Hand, A., and Fraser, F.C. Genetic counseling. The post counseling period: II. Making reproductive choices. *American Journal of Medical Genetics, 4*, 73–87 (1979).

Olshansky, S. Chronic sorrow: A response to having a mentally defective child. *Social Casework, 43*, 190–193 (1962).

Paulson, M.J., and Stone, D. Specialist-professional intervention: An expanding role in the care and treatment of the retarded and their families. In *Socio-Behavioral Studies in Mental Retardation*, R.K. Eyman, C.E. Meyers, and G. Tarjan, eds. Monograph of the AAMD, (1973), No. 1, pp. 234–240.

Richardson, S.A. Attitudes and behavior toward the physically handicapped. *Birth Defects: Original Article Series, 12*, No. 4, 15–34 (1976).

Schild, S. Psychological issues in genetic counseling of phenylketonuria. In *Genetic Counseling. Psychological Dimensions*, S. Kessler, ed. Academic Press, New York (1979), pp. 135–152.

Shear, C.S., Willman, N.S., and Nyhan, W.L. Phenylketonuria: Experience with diet and management. In *Heritable Disorders of Amino Acid Metabolism*. W.L. Nyhan, ed. Wiley, New York (1974).

Solnit, A.J., and Stark, M.H. Mourning and the birth of a defective child. *Psychoanalytic Study of the Child Journal, 16*, 523–537 (1961).

Sorenson, J.R. Some social and psychologic issues in genetic counseling. *Birth Defects: Original Article Series, 10*, No. 6, 165–199 (1974).

Spitz, R.A. Hospitalism: An inquiry into the genesis of psychiatric conditions in early childhood. In *The Psychoanalytic Study of the Child*, A. Freud, ed. International Universities Press, New York (1945), pp. 53–74.

–––. *The First Year of Life; A Psychoanalytic Study of Normal and Deviant Development of Object Relations*. International Universities Press, New York (1965).

Targum, S.D., and Weiss, J.O. A genetic disease in the family. *Psychiatric Opinion, 17*, 23–25 (1980).

Tisza, V.B., and Gumpertz, E. The parents' reaction to the birth and early care of children with cleft palate. *Pediatrics, 30*, 86–90 (1962).

Voysey, M. Impression management by parents with disabled children. *Journal of Health and Social Behavior, 13*, 80–89 (1972).

Waisbren, S.E. Parents' reactions after the birth of a developmentally disabled child. *American Journal of Mental Deficiency, 84*, 345–351 (1980).

Weiss, J.O. Social work and genetic counseling. *Social Work in Health Care, 2*, 5–12 (1976).

Whitten, C.F. Psychosocial effects of sickle cell anemia. *Archives of Internal Medicine, 133*, 681–689 (1974).

Wirls, C.J., and Plotkin, R.R. A comparison of children with cleft palate and their siblings on projective test personality factors. *Cleft Palate Journal, 8*, 399–408 (1971).

12

Emotional Impact of Hematology and Oncology Illnesses on the Child and Family

Sunny Lindamood and Fran Wiley

Recent advances in the medical treatment of childhood cancer have dramatically increased the chances of long-term survival for many children. Even in cases where cure is not possible, chances for a remission lasting for years make vigorous treatment an accepted norm. This has led to the clustering of pediatric oncology patients at major medical centers, where advanced diagnostic and treatment facilities are available. These families are doubly stressed because they are suddenly thrust into the strange atmosphere of a major medical center, often in a strange city. Even with the hopeful prognosis that can be realistically given in most cases, the emotional impact of the diagnosis of cancer is extreme and long lasting.

We have observed that most children and their families go through specific stages that are treatment related (Burgert, 1972). We will describe these stages, the tasks that must be accomplished within each stage, and the interventions that are often helpful as the children and their families learn to cope with each stage of illness and wellness.

PREDIAGNOSIS

Most patients and their families experience suspicion, fear, and anxiety during a prediagnostic phase lasting from days to weeks. Due to the insidious onset of most pediatric malignancies, parents have reported a frustrating period of suspicion without medical validation. As one articulate mother explained, "I went from doctor to doctor because I knew something was seriously wrong with my son. At the same time, I spent a great deal of energy denying that possibility. It doesn't make sense, but that's how I felt."

After receiving a firm diagnosis, parents obsessively review this period, wondering if they could have speeded up the diagnosis, if their denial delayed diagnosis and treatment, if a "better" doctor would have found it sooner, etc. Typical behavior manifests in scapegoating, hostility and rage, and feelings of guilt.

DIAGNOSIS

It is because of this experience that the phase of diagnosis is perceived by the family as one of helplessness. For many, this may be the first exposure to a large medical center. Separation from family and social supports is common. Uncertainty about the diagnosis heightens a sense of vulnerability: inability to do anything concrete for the child increases feelings of helplessness and anger.

The care of these patients requires the availability of many medical subspecialties as well as an interdisciplinary team of support personnel. At UCLA, this team includes nurses, social workers, child activity specialists, a dietician, psychologist, school teacher, physical and occupational therapists.

Even the youngest child observes that his "omnipotent" parents are not in control of this situation; his usual sources of comfort and security in times of stress are upset and unable to respond to his needs in the usual manner. His sense of vulnerability is heightened. Often, he maintains a stoic facade, asking no questions, for fear of further upsetting his parents. This response is anticipated, and play therapists become involved in helping the patient express—through play, drawing, or words—his many conflicting feelings.

We emphasize the idea of "open information" from the first day (Baker, 1976). We share the diagnosis of a specific malignancy with the child and his entire family (Lavigne and Ryan, 1979). Most parents find this difficult and want to withhold information in order to protect the child. It is our task at this point to work with the child's parents to help them understand why it is so important for their child to fully understand what is going to be happening to him, and why (Binger, 1969). This is usually accomplished within hours or, at most, days. We emphasize that cancer is not a bad word and purposefully use correct terminology to give a sense of mastery and to demystify an alien environment.

In addition to repeated conferences with the child and family during the diagnostic period, we also give concrete information in the form of pamphlets and books. The American Cancer Society and the National Cancer Institute are good sources, both for English and Spanish versions. It is important to assess the age-appropriateness of written materials and to use them as teaching aids, not substitutes for individual teaching about the illness and its treatment (Baker, 1976).

We arrange one-to-one contacts with patients who are already undergoing treatment for a similar illness, as most families want to speak with someone who has first-hand experience and has gained mastery of a similar situation. This is valid not only for the child and his parents, but also the siblings. We also encourage the patient and family to keep a written record of what is occurring—and in their record, to write down any questions or problems so they remember to discuss them with us.

INITIAL TREATMENT

Once a diagnosis is made, the phase of initial treatment begins. This is usually a lengthy and arduous time during which the reality of cancer becomes physically apparent to all those involved with the sick child. The major task of this stage is coping, with as little chaos as possible. Any preexisting psychosocial stress in the family, such as a divorce, marital upset, or adolescent acting out, is bound to be exacerbated by a diagnosis of cancer (Lansky et al., 1978). A thorough psychosocial assessment is necessary to predict which families will need intensive intervention. While all families will need crisis intervention in the beginning, we have found that the following situations usually warrant more intensive psychotherapy: denial by the patient or his parents of the reality or severity of the illness; inability of the parents to communicate about the disease; refusal, by the patient or his parents, to accept treatment; abject mistrust of all medical personnel; exacerbation of preexisting, or initiation of, substance abuse; and, severe, debilitating depression (Stebbens and Laskari, 1974). Depending on the resources of the treatment facility and the proximity of the family to it, intensive psychotherapy can be arranged either in the home community or at the treatment center.

It is necessary during this stage to reteach much of the information that was given in the diagnostic period. Many parents recall "hearing the word 'cancer' and nothing after that." The patients come to the clinic and realize that pain is to become a part of their life. The children gradually learn to cope with painful procedures. This is facilitated in a variety of ways: play therapy is used; relaxation techniques and guided imagery are taught to help in dealing with nausea and pain. In addition, both the children and families make friends in the clinic. These relationships become very supportive.

In one situation, Suzette, a four-year-old patient being treated for relapse of Wilms' tumor was able to help a seven-year-old newly diagnosed with the same illness. Suzette met Alice in the clinic playroom. Their discussion revealed that Alice was terrified of injections. Suzette offered to help. She taught Alice a diversionary counting game and invited the new patient to watch her receive her own injection. From this beginning, the children have become friends and continue to be mutually supportive during painful procedures.

It is also during the stage of initial treatment that we focus on the patient's siblings. Largely forgotten entities in the diagnostic phase, they need explanations about what is happening to their brother or sister. It is common for siblings to feel resentment. We find that including them in the care of their sibling, explaining medical information, and acknowledging their special concerns does much to foster good family relations (Lavigne and Ryan, 1979). Magical thinking also needs to be addressed. Siblings, as well as patients, often think they caused the illness and that they can control the outcome.

During this phase, the parents' marriage is predictably stressed (Lansky et al., 1978). Preventive counselling is done to warn of possible problems and pitfalls and to give reassurance that help with these problems is available. It is important to overtly encourage the fathers to stay involved in the care of the patient, to come to the clinic with the child if at all possible. Severe stress can occur when the mother becomes sole caretaker and thereby is indirectly held responsible for complications and outcome of treatment.

Most parents become involved in the parents' group during this stage (Lindamood et al., 1979). This forum provides opportunity for shared information about problems and their solutions, supportive therapy, and formal lectures on topics of mutual interest (e.g., nutrition for the cancer patient, or how to discipline a child with a low platelet count). The group meets in the evenings, further encouraging the fathers to attend.

REMISSION

The third stage of the cancer experience is that of remission. This is a happy time, when the child and his family feel that things may return to normal. The task during this period seems to be adaptive denial. When the family is not at the clinic for treatment, the members want to forget about the disease and its ramifications. This is acknowledged, and therapeutic interventions focus on how well the family has adapted to its situation. We encourage the patients and families to help newer patients, by talking and by example. It is very therapeutic to realize that you have mastered a situation enough to be able to help someone else with the same problems you were having only a few months previously. "Old Timer" parents offer to go to the home of a new patient to discuss issues about the illness. Teenage amputees offer to help teach new patients how to deal with prostheses. Siblings counsel other siblings about surviving with less of Mom's attention.

Remission is also the time when the family has the luxury of worrying about the things that seemed too trivial to consider during diagnosis and initial treatment: for the parents, the reality of financial changes, such as the mother having to quit her job or the father having to keep an unfulfilling job to guarantee continuing insurance coverage; fear that future children may also have a malignancy; the sadness that there may be no grandchildren; the worry that the patient's siblings will permanently resent him and all the attention that he has received; the realization that the marriage has had to take second place to the illness. For the patient, there are fears of returning to school: how the other children will react; the possibility of being ridiculed about changed appearance. For older patients concerns center around body image, dating, sterility, employability, and secondary malignancy. The psychosocial issues often take precedence over medical issues during remission, and therapeutic intervention is focused on patient and family counseling.

RELAPSE

Unfortunately, many children do suffer a recurrence of their malignancy. At relapse, the task of family, patient, and staff is coping with a new crisis. This crisis in many ways mimics the diagnostic phase; the family reexperiences shock, disbelief, guilt, and anger. The interventions are also similar to those of the diagnostic phase. The patient and family need permission and time to grieve. They need new, concrete information, repeated as necessary. Before they are able to make appropriate decisions about further treatment or palliation, they need support and understanding. The denial, so well developed during remission, makes it difficult to move quickly. The parents frequently describe a loss of naive innocence as the possibility/probability that their child may not be cured gradually seeps in. There is a gradual change from hope for a cure to hope for some good time.

An added stress occurs because family members work through this crisis at different rates and may not be able to offer each other much support.

The "not to tell" issue usually surfaces again. Besides the obvious motivation of wanting to protect the child from painful knowledge, the parents may exhibit a good deal of projection. When they say, "I'm afraid he will give up," they often mean, "I am afraid I want to give up" or, "I cannot tolerate starting all over again." Subterfuge is again discouraged and clarification provided, because good parent-child communication is vital during this decision-making time. In reality, even the youngest patient is fully aware that something is wrong and is relieved to be able to discuss it.

In contrast to the diagnostic crises, the incapacitating shock and disorganization experienced are usually of shorter duration. The family has learned coping mechanisms and has developed support systems during the treatment phase. They are comfortable with and trust the staff. It is important to be aware of staff reactions to the diagnosis of relapse. By now, the whole team has come to know the family well and also has a clearer understanding than the family of the implications of a relapse. The disappointment and grief felt by the staff cannot be discounted and must be dealt with before a truly therapeutic milieu can be reestablished.

Though another remission is frequently achieved, the knowledge that relapse has occurred changes the future outlook. Relatively soon after the diagnosis of relapse most families again use adaptive denial in order to function. However, they realize that their chances for cure have dramatically decreased.

DYING

When the child enters a dying trajectory, the task is letting go. If done prematurely, this may lead to abandonment of the child. The staff can provide much support to help the family through this period. Most parents and older patients want to know specifically what will happen and how, but they are often afraid to broach these subjects. Concrete explanations of the physiological and psychological processes are a good starting point. The real goal is to provide for the best quality of life possible in the circumstances present. In order to maintain open communication, additional efforts must be made to support the siblings and extended family. The family needs an advocate in making decisions. They must be secure that all decisions are in the child's best interest. Many families rethink issues of alternative forms of therapy as they review events. We acknowledge this need and prevent much family disruption by understanding their desperation, and reassuring them that their child has had and will continue to have the best possible care. When further consultation is appropriate or needed by the family to assure them that no stone has been left unturned, we help arrange it. The act of offering to arrange consultation is in itself reassuring.

The concept of home death has gained popularity over the years, but it is not appropriate for every family. The therapeutic goal is to help the family and patient decide what is best for them without placing value judgments on their decision. These decisions may change frequently.

The key to the success of a home care program is 24-hour access to a supportive person who knows the child well and the opportunity for readmission to the hospital at any time. Maternal exhaustion, reassessment of pain management, or a transfusion are all appropriate reasons for a short hospital admission. In order to assure the best possible quality of life, multimodality individualized pain management is vital whether the child is hospitalized or at home.

While the focus of attention is certainly the dying child, consideration must be given to the survivors. The thrust of psychotherapuetic intervention must be in helping the family master the loss and go on. They need to feel that they did everything possible for the child and that they made the right decisions for the right reasons.

Much integrative work must be done after the death of the patient. Following the death, we continue contact with the whole family. We encourage them to return to the treatment center to discuss autopsy findings and ask any questions. An assessment is made of the need for further psychiatric intervention. Siblings have many concerns and fears at this time but are often hesitant to discuss them with their parents, who are obviously in pain. Parents may be either unaware of or unable to deal with these issues.

Every parent appreciates letters from the physician and other staff expressing sorrow and acknowledgment of their loss. These letters are cherished, reread, and saved.

Lack of skilled bereavement counseling is a problem in many communities. Bereavement groups are one effective self-help modality that is becoming more widely known and supported throughout the country.

SURVIVING PATIENTS

A significant proportion of pediatric cancer patients never suffer a relapse and go on to become long-term survivors. These children have very special needs, and the practicing clinician must be ready to deal with these patients in growing numbers.

The emotional theme that pervades the termination of treatment is ambivalence. Younger children are happy to have fewer painful experiences, but most parents and older patients describe a sense of surprise at the ambivalence felt. They have counted the days to termination but now realize that they have come to regard the treatment as a magical way to ward off disaster. Ending treatment is giving up the "security blanket" and becoming vulnerable again.

Frequently voiced concerns include apologies for needing continuing support and anxieties about follow-up outside the treatment center. There is a fear of loss of the supportive community of staff and other families at the center. We confront this overtly, acknowledging the concerns and assuring our availability. We emphasize our own trust and confidence in the community physician and assure the availability of the treatment team to him as well.

Even if the child has been cured of the childhood malignancy, there is a loss of innocence that reawakens at each new crisis. The usually vague symptoms present at the initial diagnosis of cancer are all too common in the human experience. An occasional fever, swollen node, or bruise are not minor concerns ever again.

The normal adolescent struggles for emancipation may be exaggerated in an effort to combat the overprotectiveness that most parents continue to demonstrate toward the patient. Concerns about the ability or advisability of procreation occur years later when marriage is contemplated. The patient and his family frequently return for advice and support about these issues, and are encouraged to do so.

Many of the families who have finished the treatment assume the role of old graduate. Their active involvement in the parents' group and counseling of new families gives a needed opportunity to experience altruism and a feeling of repayment.

CONCLUSION

In summary, the experience of childhood cancer has been described as occurring in specific stages of prediagnosis, diagnosis, initial treatment, remission, relapse, death, or survival. The emotional impact of this experience on the child, his family, and community is significant and longlasting. Whatever the medical outcome, families facing these predictable crises need skilled supportive care. The continuing consideration of the psychosocial needs of these families is a major component of good treatment.

REFERENCES

Baker, L. *You and Leukemia.* Mayo Comprehensive Cancer Center, Rochester, Minn. (1976).

Binger, C.M. Childhood leukemia: Emotional impact on patient and family. *New England Journal of Medicine, 280,* 414 (1969).

Burgert, O.E. Emotional impact of childhood acute leukemia. *Mayo Clinic Proceedings, 47,* 273-277 (1972).

Lansky, S.B., Cairns, N.U., Itassanein, R., Wehr, J., and Lowman, J.T. Childhood cancer: Parental discord and divorce. *Pediatrics, 62,* 184-188 (1978).

Lavigne, J., and Ryan, M. Psychologic adjustment of siblings of children with chronic illness. *Pediatrics, 63,* 4 (1979).

Lindamood, M., Wiley, F.M., Schmidt, M.L., and Rhein, M.J. Groups for bereaved parents—how they can help. *Journal of Family Practice, 9,* 1027-1033 (1979).

Stebbens, J.A., and Lascari, A.D. Psychological followup of families with childhood malignancy. *Journal of Clinical Psychology, 30,* 394 (1974).

13

The Psychosocial Aspects of Hemophilia

Shelby L. Dietrich, Margaret A. Jaffe, and Margaret K. Reed

Hemophilia is a term applied to genetically transmitted congenital coagulation deficiencies, of which the most common are hemophilia A (classic hemophilia, or factor VIII deficiency) and hemophilia B (Christmas disease, or factor IX deficiency). Both of these types of hemophilia are genetically transmitted as X-linked recessive disorders; thus they are clinically manifested in the male, while the mother and other female relatives are carriers. Although no definite "cure" exists for hemophilia, the development of plasma clotting factor concentrate in the past 15 years has changed the medical treatment dramatically and consequently improved the physical and emotional well-being of families and patients with hemophilia (Boone, 1976).

The diagnosis of hemophilia, usually confirmed in the child's first year of life, brings inevitable stress to the parents and the other family members. A great deal of time and sensitivity are required to assist the parents with acceptance of the diagnosis of hemophilia and understanding the genetic transmission, clinical manifestations, and treatment available to their child. Approximately one-third of newly diagnosied hemophilia cases will be found in families *without* a known family history of hemophilia; these cases are regarded as new mutations. Regardless of family history, it is essential to explore parental feelings about the genetics of hemophilia and to provide appropriate psychotherapeutic services to facilitate resolution of maternal guilt and anxiety about transmitting this disease. This early counseling is a difficult but very important task, and its handling may set the tone for the long-term relationship with the family and the child. Ideally, the comprehensive hemophilia treatment center will be adequately staffed with mental health professionals (i.e., clinical social worker, psychologist, psychiatrist) who can assess parental readiness and offer in-depth counseling appropriately timed to meet the needs of individual families (Hilgartner, 1979). Basically, the family may be assured that the child will have normal growth and development, will have no more than the usual illnesses of childhood, and will lead a *relatively* normal life, contingent upon adequate medical treatment as well as parental attitudes and understanding. Questions of transmission or of the genetic status of the mother or other female relatives should be referred to a hematologist or knowledgeable geneticist.

The "toddler" years are particularly difficult ones for the parents of the child goes through the normal developmental stages of exploration of the environment and increasing physical activity. At times bleeding episodes may become more frequent. Parents must be informed and counseled as to the importance of consistent and firm discipline combined with the opportunity to let the child explore a "safe" environment with as few restrictions as are necessary. Close relationships with a pediatrician and the hemophilia treatment center staff will facilitate medical and psychosocial care.

At age three to four, preschool experience may be very valuable for the child, teaching him socialization, providing group experience, and providing the child with an opportunity to begin to learn his own limitations and set his limits. When the child is ready for entrance into kindergarten, he may enter a regular school and usually does not need the services of a school for the physically handicapped. Parental problems during the early childhood years usually fluctuate between overpermissiveness and overrestriction. The precept that the child must learn by experience *what activities are safe for him* is axiomatic.

Both the parents and the child must learn to accept the inevitable need for intravenous treatment with plasma concentrate. Even a frightened two-year-old can be reassured during a somewhat painful treatment by letting him sit on his mother's lap and assist wherever possible in his own treatment, even if only by applying a Band-Aid. A certain tolerance and acceptance of pain should also be developed. For the child with severe hemophilia, a program of treatment at home with the parent or caretaker administering the concentrate may be feasible by age four to six. Supervised self-infusion has been enthusiastically, if not overwhelmingly, accepted by most patients with hemophilia because of the freedom from the hospital and the relatively normal lifestyle that it affords.

Adolescence is a particularly difficult time for all parents and children. It is the final step between dependence and independence. It is during this time that most people with hemophilia learn self-infusion and are given the responsibility for self-care. At this time, the overprotective parents become concerned about their child's future and its limited options, and the child tries in vain to remain cared for and protected. The overpermissive parents develop very real fears about the high-risk activities in which their son partakes, not understanding why he chooses motorcycle trail racing as his testing area. Somewhere there is a middle ground, but the learning does not start at age 12 or 13. It begins when the child is small and is learning alternatives.

When discussing handicaps, much emphasis is placed on limitations or setting limits. It is important that this be placed in perspective. As a child grows, he learns about his capabilities. He finds that he is good in mathematics or shop or sports. Thus he gets positive reinforcement for these "specialities," perhaps eventually turning these skills into a profession (i.e., teacher or computer programmer, mechanic or carpenter, physical education instructor or professional athlete). But in each of these cases, the implication is that there are other areas in which the individual cannot perform as successfully. The adolescent who excels in math may be uncoordinated; the one in shop may have an inability to retain memorized facts; and the one in sports, who catches a football with such grace, may be unable to saw a piece of wood without cutting himself. Although these areas of "weakness" (not being perfect) may result in moments of disappointment, the individual usually moves on from this and "does his thing." His limitations are forgotten—or at least put aside for a while—and his emphasis is returned to his capabilities.

Every person, child or adult, has capabilities and limitations. Hopefully, one will continue to learn about these through one's whole life. And so in this very real sense, each of us is handicapped and each individual with a physical handicap has capabilities.

It is these capabilities that must be found, tapped, and encouraged. To put this into perspective, a child with hemophilia can have as full a future as anyone else, if he is given the same respect and provided with the same guidelines (expectations) according to his capabilities (not his limitations) as any other child. If this occurs, he will then have more alternatives than he will have time to explore.

The reader may consult several available references for a more detailed explanation of the medical and psychosocial aspects of hemophilia. A network of federally funded comprehensive treatment centers also exists, and the National Hemophilia Foundation, 19 West 34th Street, New York, New York, 10001, has available a geographic directory of services as well as a number of helpful publications for the parent, patient, or professional.

REFERENCES

Boone, D.C. *Comprehensive Management of Hemophilia.* F.A. Davis, Philadelphia (1976).
Hilgartner, M. Managing the child with hemophilia. *Pediatric Annals, 8,* 68–84 (1979).

14

Psychological Considerations for the
Cleft Palate Clinic and Team

Yoshio Setoguchi and Patricia DuPont-Norton

The concept of a multidisciplinary approach to the care of a child with a physical handicap has been advocated for many years. In no other condition is this type of health delivery more important than in the management of a child who has a cleft lip and palate or cleft palate.

Over the years the actual clinical implication of the multidisciplinary or team approach to treatment has taken different forms, and one approach is that which is used at the UCLA Craniofacial Anomalies Clinic. The three most important underlying principles that have led to the procedures used by our clinic are: (1) the need for individual evaluation by each team member who will have a role in the care of the patient, (2) the need for these same members to meet to discuss their findings and recommendations to determine the long- and short-term goals for the patient, and (3) the inclusion of the patient and/or parents as part of the team in finalizing the treatment program plan.

Most cleft palate or craniofacial anomaly clinics (the term *orofacial* is also used) are composed of a plastic surgeon, orthodontist, pediatrician, speech pathologist, audiologist, otolaryngologist, social worker, psychologist, prosthodontist, pedodontist, geneticist, radiologist, and oral surgeon. Many clinics also utilize the services of a dental radiologist, neurosurgeon, ophthalmologist, and psychiatrist. As can be seen, this is a large group of specialists, and for them to function effectively as a team, a coordinator is essential.

The coordinator can come from any of the aforementioned disciplines. The most important functions of the coordinator are to arrange for the various evaluations that the patient requires, conduct team meetings to determine the goals and priorities of treatment, and to discuss with the patient and/or family the findings and decisions of the team. The coordinator should also be available for discussions with the family if there are additional questions or concerns about the treatment plan.

The intake procedure at UCLA is similar to that of most clinics. Referrals are received from a variety of sources, including those from private physicians, school nurses, speech pathologists or clinics, parents, friends, and frequently from Crippled (California) Children Services (CCS). When a referral is received, the family is contacted by the clinic secretary to obtain the basic information about the patient, including diagnosis and past treatment. The secretary also describes the type of clinic we have and the procedures that will be involved during the initial evaluation. Because our initial evaluation is very comprehensive and time consuming, this explanation and description of the clinic often prevents misconceptions and complaints that could arise in the future.

Next, the family is sent an appointment for the initial evaluation, together with a brief printed description of our clinic composition and a review of the clinic's procedures. The first appointment scheduled is an office visit for a pediatric and social work evaluation. The social worker sees the patient first to obtain pertinent information regarding:

1. The reason for the referral to our clinic.
2. The expectations of the patient and family regarding the evaluation
3. The resources available to the patient and/or family to follow through with treatment recommendations
4. The psychosocial structure of the family and the effects to date of the craniofacial anomaly on the patient and family

It is important to obtain a complete medical history and physical examination. This is done by the team pediatrician. Following the examination, the pediatrician determines those consultations with other specialists that are needed to obtain a complete evaluation of the child's medical and dental needs.

At UCLA the patient and family are scheduled for from two to six additional visits. The second patient visit is in the clinic setting. The following team disciplines are available to evaluate the patient: genetics, pedodontics, orthodontics, plastic surgery, oral surgery, and prosthodontics. X-Ray facilities are available for cephalometrics, panorex, and skull series if needed. Subsequent appointments may include ENT, audiology, speech pathology, ophthalmology, and neurosurgery.

When all of the evaluations recommended by the team coordinator have been completed, the patient is scheduled for presentation at the next team conference. At the conference, all of the various evaluations are presented and discussed. After the findings and recommendations of each team member have been presented, priorities of treatment as well as short- and long-term goals are formulated.

The team coordinator then meets with the patient and family to discuss the recommendations and to examine their feelings regarding the recommendations. Questions that they ask or concerns expressed, are answered.

Ours is primarily a consultation clinic; therefore, once the treatment recommendations have been made and the patient has accepted them, the actual treatment is usually referred to a qualified local practitioner. In planning an ongoing treatment program, the team should consider such factors as the length of treatment, frequency of appointments, financial status of the family, the employment status of both parents, and transportation capabilities. It is for these reasons that clinics at major academic institutions provide actual treatment procedures to only 50-60 percent of the patients who are seen for consultation.

The surgical, dental, and speech treatment of the cleft lip and palate patient can usually be handled in a very efficient manner by private practitioners, without the benefit of a clinic team. However, it is in the area of psychosocial needs of the patients that the team approach is superior to the limited method of treatment.

The need for psychosocial treatment begins at the birth of the child. It is therefore important for members of the team, usually the pediatrician and social worker, to see the child and parents as soon after the birth as possible, to enable them to deal with the multitude of feelings and questions the family may have.

The birth of a child is usually a time of joy and celebration. The parents have prepared for the many things they will do with this new family member. However, the birth of a "handicapped" child destroys many of those plans. The initial reactions of the parents are sadness, feelings of isolation, embarrassment, and feelings of failure or inadequacy. The initial period of shock is usually followed by anger, guilt, frustration, and depression.

The practitioner working with the family must realize and convey to the parents that these are normal reactions and that they need to work through their feelings. Inability to accept these feelings and to deal with them in a positive manner will later lead to overprotection or rejection of the child. The neonatal period is the ideal time for intervention, since the parents have not had time to develop unhealthy defense mechanisms, and other people have not had an opportunity to give them very much misinformation. Misinformation and misleading information can come from well-meaning but often incorrectly informed family members, from friends, and even from the hospital staff.

Once the initial shock has been dealt with, the parents usually have many serious questions pertaining to the child's condition. The four most frequently heard at our clinic are:

1. Why did this happen?
2. Is this hereditary?
3. What can be done? Can anything be done right away?
4. What about our baby's future? Will he/she be normal?

The most difficult question to answer is the first one. Many parents are looking for someone or something to blame. This may be each other, relatives, or even the physicians. Displacement of anger is a defense mechanism by which the parents try to deal with their feelings of hopelessness and helplessness. The object of this displacement is often inappropriate, but unless the pediatrician and social worker are aware that these feelings do occur they may respond to the anger with their own hostilities.

Since the presence of a cleft lip and palate has hereditary implications, it is important to discuss this with the parents. Referral to a geneticist in the neonatal period is usually unnecessary unless the infant presents other anomalies. But the parents should have a simple, brief, initial explanation of the genetic possibilities. Terms such as *polygenic* or *multifactoral* mean little to the parents and may further confuse and depress them. During this period of adjustment the parents do not need more unknowns and problems. Later, when the family has adjusted to the initial shock of having a child with a cleft lip and palate, more thorough genetic counseling may be helpful.

In some cases there is already a known family history of the condition. In such cases there is no question of who is to blame. However, this knowledge in itself may be a problem, as one of the parents may have been the prime motivator for having the child, believing he could "beat the odds." When the child is born with cleft lip and/or palate there may easily be considerable guilt felt by that parent.

Although the parents may not have completely worked out their feelings, they are usually still anxious to learn about what can be done for the child. As soon as possible, the physician should inform the family that much can be done to *decrease*—not correct—the appearance created by the anomalies. Each area of treatment, such as plastic surgery, orthodontics, otology, and speech, must be discussed in a simple but clear manner. Initially, the family is not interested in the technical details of the treatment, but they are interested in the timing of the treatment and the ultimate prognosis. The key to successful intervention is to "not overwhelm" the family.

Once they know that treatment is available, many parents ask if their child will be able to lead a normal life. Generally, however, they are more concerned about medical problems than about the psychosocial development of the child. If defense mechanisms are observed that could adversely affect the child's psychosocial development, intervention should be introduced. Discussion with the parents about their attitudes and feelings can be helpful, and the services of a parent group can be beneficial. Some of the family's questions regarding the results of treatment; the effect of the deformities on peer relationships; and problems of the child in coping with teasing, adjustment to school, and so on can be answered effectively by qualified parents who have already had the experience of raising a child with a cleft lip and/or palate.

The child should be given a complete medical and dental examination. Although the need for the latter is sometimes questioned, since dentition is not usually seen in an infant, it is important to get a thorough assessment of the oral structures, particularly as related to the cleft.

After the examinations and evaluations have been completed, the parents need to be told in a simple and concise manner the extent of the child's problems and the general treatment procedures recommended. The physician should recognize that, because of the emotional status of the parents, much of the information will be missed or misunderstood. The parents should be encouraged to ask questions, and the physician should answer these questions even if it means reiterating many of the important points about the diagnosis and treatment.

Feeding the infant who has a cleft lip and palate is the first problem the parents will encounter. There are inherent mechanical difficulties for the infant to sustain a good sucking action. If sustained sucking is the only difficulty, satisfactory oral intake can be achieved through the use of special nipples, bottles, and positioning. At UCLA we try to minimize the logistic problems for the family by recommending a preemie nipple with an enlarged opening (corsshatched) on a regular bottle. The infant is then held in an upright position and otherwise fed in the usual manner. Breast feeding is *not* impossible, but it is a little more difficult than with a normal child. Breast feeding can be accomplished by a determined mother and supportive, knowledgeable medical staff. Excellent articles are available on this subject and will therefore not be discussed in this chapter (Grady, 1977; Paradise and McWilliams, 1974; Pashayan and McNab, 1979).

If, after making adjustments for the mechanical difficulties the infant is still having difficulty in obtaining satisfactory oral intake, two other problems may exist. There may be additional physical conditions affecting the child. If the mother has not properly understood the description of the infant's condition, she may be afraid the baby will choke or that she will hurt it. If her feelings about the physical abnormalities have not been worked through, she may want to get each feeding over with in a hurry. In either case, the infant will not have had the time or opportunity to obtain sufficient nutrition. When feeding problems persist after the mechanical reasons have been compensated for, the possibility of the mother's emotional stresses needs to be explored.

Now, to take the child home! Most parents feel safe and emotionally protected during the postpartum hospitalization. However, that supportive, protected environment does not usually extend beyond the confines of the hospital. Thus parents must be given every opportunity to ventilate fears, anxieties, and frustrations during the hospitalization period so that they will be prepared to deal with any unpleasantries later from uninformed and often insensitive persons. Such preparation can help the family to deal constructively with their social environment and avoid being emotionally damaged by negative experiences.

Parents need reassurance that they are adequate and that they are able and capable of properly caring for their disabled child. However, they must clearly understand what is expected of them in terms of the "in-home" care of the child after discharge from the hospital.

With this understanding, preparation for surgery should also be introduced, with careful emphasis placed on a time frame. Discussion of the anticipated surgery often provides an element of optimism for the family, as it indicates that, indeed, something can and will be done for the child but within appropriate stages of the child's growth and development.

Although feeding problems are common during the period preceding surgical closure of the lip (at around three to four months of age) and the palate (at approximately 18 months of age), most parents do quite well. However, they may frequently express the feeling that they are looking forward to the impending surgery and that they are emotionally prepared for it. Once surgery is actually scheduled, however, and the child is admitted to the hospital, we have found that even the most prepared parents need additional supportive contact. It has proven to be helpful to parents to have the pediatric coordinator and/or social worker make frequent contacts with the parents, particularly on the day of surgery and throughout the child's hospital stay. The most frequent questions raised are, in effect:

1. Will my child look significantly different?
2. If so, will I be able to accept this new appearance?
3. What might go wrong during surgery that I may have previously failed to ask?
4. Is my child going to be in much pain?
5. Will I be pleased with my child's appearance?

Appearance! Ours is a society that places a great deal of importance on facial and physical appearance. The birth of a child with a cleft lip and palate brings to the forefront just how much facial appearance is valued. Not only must parents deal with questions, stares, and comments from others, but they must eventually deal with their own child when he begins to ask, "What happened to my face? Why don't I look like everyone else?"

The face in our society is often viewed as a "reflection of the self," but the face of the person with a cleft lip and palate is so often seen as the only reflection, and the self remains hidden and depressed, lacking self-esteem. Society so often refuses to see beyond the scar or to listen beyond the often hypernasal quality of speech to hear what the person with the cleft lip and palate has to say.

Since so much emphasis is placed on the face in reference to a person's appearance, it is encouraging to note that major developments are being made in the area of plastic/corrective surgery, which offers hope to patients and their families that, indeed, much can be done to improve the facial appearance of persons with cleft lip and palate. Such persons can be given considerable assurance that they will eventually be able to go forth in a society where normal facial appearance plays a significant role in the development of self-esteem.

REFERENCES

Grady, E. Breastfeeding the baby with a cleft of the soft palate: Success and its benefits. *Clinical Pediatrics, 16,* 978–981 (1977).

Paradise, J.L., and McWilliams, B.J. Simplified feeder for infants with cleft palate. *Pediatrics, 53,* 566–568 (1974).

Pashayan, H.M., and McNab, M. Simplified method of feeding infants born with cleft palate with or without cleft lip. *American Journal of Diseases of Children, 133,* 145–147 (1979).

Psychological Considerations in the
Spinal Defects and Meningomyelocele Clinic

Shirley T. Whiteman and Wendy S. Feldman

Until 25 years ago, few babies born with spina bifida or myelodysplasia survived beyond infancy or early childhood. Today it is possible for many such children not only to grow into adulthood but to live productive lives.

Spina bifida is a disease entity that includes a group of developmental defects of the spinal column in which there is a failure of fusion of vertebral arches with or without protrusion and dysplasia of the spinal cord and its membranes. In the embryological development of this birth defect, there is seen in the fetus a failure of proper closure of the neural tube. This developmental defect occurs on the 25th to the 29th day of gestation (Patten, 1953).

This occurs in the midline of the back and includes a defect of the vertebral arches occurring posteriorly in any part of the spinal column from the base of the brain at the back of the neck caudally to the sacrum. Usually quite evident at the time of birth, a visible swelling can be seen on the baby's back. Most commonly this presents as a fluid-filled, membranous sac, and less frequently as a solid tissue mass. In the central aspect of this lesion can often be visualized the neural plate, or that part of the neural tissue that fails to develop properly, and overlying this sac there is often a very faint network of neural tissue evident.

Neural tube defect is a broader term that includes anencephaly or brain involvement and spina bifida or spinal cord involvement. A variety of defects can occur. Spina bifida occulta, in which there is a lack of fusion of the vertebral arches without any cystic distension of the meninges, is a common finding even in normal children and is of no genetic or statistical significance in the study of this group of patients. Likewise, anencephaly, which is a cephalad neural plate defect, is of importance in the prenatal detection of neural tube defects but not significant in the overall study and treatment of the spina bifida patient, since anencephaly is not compatible with life.

For practical purposes, spina bifida or spina bifida cystica may be divided into two categories:

1. Meningocele, in which there is a lack of fusion of the vertebral arches with cystic distension of the meninges, but absence of myelodysplasia

of the spinal cord and absence of any neurological signs, such as paraplegia, incontinence, etc. This group of patients still has continuity of
the neural lesion to the ventricles of the brain and may develop hydrocephalus.
2. Myelomeningocele, in which there is a lack of fusion of the vertebral
   arches, cystic distension of the meninges, myelodysplasia of the spinal
   cord, and neurological signs that become evident at the level of the
   lesion and caudally.

INCIDENCE AND GENETICS

Neural tube defects are among the most common major congenital malformations. The natural incidence of spina bifida varies in different parts of the world
and shows a range of 0.3 per thousand births in Japan to over four per thousand
births in some parts of the British Isles. In the United States the number of spina
bifida births has been slowly declining, and in most studies is usually stated as
two per thousand live births. There were peaks of incidence in the 1920s and in
the 1950s, especially in England, with the incidence highest in Ireland and
Northern Wales. Studies in the United States have shown an incidence slightly
lower than in Europe. Ethnic variations are reported, and there is a slight preponderance of females over males: about 1.3 to 1.0 in most series (Brocklehurst,
1976).

A positive family history has been obtained about 10 percent of the time.
The recurrence rate when there is an affected child is just over five percent.
After two affected infants, the chances of yet another are between 10 and 15
percent (Brocklehurst, 1976).

The cause of spina bifida has not been determined. The method of transmission genetically is referred to as multifactorial inherited predisposition. This
simply implies both a familial and an environmental etiology. Despite many
theories, many reports, and many studies, there is no consistent etiologic factor
known.

Recently, considerable headway has been made in prenatal detection by
working with alpha-fetoprotein (AFP) levels in the maternal blood and in the
fluid obtained from amniocentesis. A neural tube defect in the fetus is accompanied by increased plasma levels of alpha-fetoprotein in the period between 16
and 24 weeks of gestation. In a screening procedure the maternal AFP level can
be measured. If abnormally elevated, amniocentesis studies can be utilized to
confirm the diagnosis. Here, too, there is an elevation of alpha-fetoprotein.
Further diagnostic studies, such as fetoscopy or ultrasound, are then utilized to
confirm the presence of a neural tube defect (Crandall, 1981).

What problems will the baby have? Most evident at the time of birth and in
subsequent development of the child is the problem of paralysis, the degree of

which is usually determined by the level of the lesion. Therefore, at a high level or thoracic lesion, the child will be paralyzed below the waist, with all the related complications of such paralysis (lack of sensation to touch and to heat; lack of mobility; inability to ambulate independently; and a more subtle, but serious, complication of such paralysis: incontinence of urine and feces). In the newborn this is overlooked and does not present an acute problem, but by the time the child approaches two, three, or four years of age, and especially by the time the child reaches school age, this becomes a much more acute problem. Many orthopedic deformities will result from lack of proper enervation to the lower extremities. Muscle imbalances will occur, and joints will sublux or dislocate. The child will often be born with club foot deformities of varying degrees. Ironically, the baby with the lower-level lesion will often walk independently, even though there is a lack of sensation in and deformities of the feet. Yet as this child grows older and into adulthood, devastating complications related to foot deformities can occur because of poor skin care, ulcers, and osteomyelitis, and, in a few cases, the damage is severe enough to necessitate amputation.

In addition to the paraplegia and incontinence, a further difficulty—hydrocephalus—occurs in about 50 percent of the patients. In some cases of hydrocephalus there is an abnormally rapid and excessive enlargement of the head due to distension of the ventricular cavities with cerebrospinal fluid. The fluid is accumulated because of anatomical and physiological changes, which interfere with the circulation and absorption of the spinal fluid. This complication of the circulation of spinal fluid occurs because of a distortion of the base of the brain and lower brain stem, a condition called the Arnold-Chiari malformation, or sometimes because of another defect called aqueduct stenosis. In the majority of patients, problems of hydrocephalus become evident quite early, either *in utero* or shortly after birth, or after the back lesion has been repaired. Only rarely does hydrocephalus first manifest itself in the older child or young adult. On rare occasions, there are other associated birth defects, some common to the spina bifida child and some completely sporadic. Therefore, all of these factors of the spina bifida baby must be taken into consideration in the initial discussions with the new parents.

MENTAL CAPACITY

Much of the literature related to the survival and intellectual development of children born with spina bifida cites a large number of mentally retarded (Black, 1979). However, as with any major defect, just as life expectancy is improving day by day with utilization of advanced medical care, so is the prevention of mental retardation, since a large group of the mentally retarded children have been those with more advanced hydrocephalus and more complications related to the hydrocephalus. Surgical shunting to prevent progression of hydrocephalus can salvage brain function in many affected children.

OTHER ANOMALIES

The majority of other anomalies are usually confined to those systems already involved with myelodysplasia sequelae, such as central nervous, genitourinary, and musculoskeletal systems. Twelve percent of the patients may demonstrate central nervous system anomalies at birth; these include not only hydrocephalus, but also facial palsy, caudocranial dysostosis, and cleft palate. The latter two were only single occurrences in a large study of almost 500 patients (Banta et al., 1976). Seven percent had other genitourinary anomalies not related to the neurogenic bladder or paralysis sequelae such as horseshoe kidney, solitary kidney, or uteropelvic junction obstruction, or displaced or pelvic kidney, or duplication of either one or both renal systems. Nineteen percent had musculoskeletal deformities that probably were directly related to the degree or the level of the paralysis, the most prevalent being club foot deformity. The incidence of other system anomalies was infrequent. Two percent had gastrointestinal anomalies such as pyloric stenosis. Less than one percent had circulatory system problems such as congenital heart disease. Five percent had subsequent ENT anomalies, usually laryngeal paralysis of some type; these were rarely present at birth, but became apparent within the first year of life. Strabismus, too, was rarely present at birth, but became apparent in 20 percent of the patients by the time they reached school age (Banta et al., 1976).

Of particular importance is the ENT problem of laryngeal paralysis, seen at any time within the first few years but usually within the first few months of life. The most common is the closed type of laryngeal paralysis, or vocal cord paralysis, wherein the infant develops stridor, often to the point of needing tracheostomy. Much less frequent is the open type of paralysis, where there is recurrent aspiration because of poor swallowing coordination, causing repeated pneumonia, which is often life-threatening, as well as leading to failure to thrive. This group of children not only require tracheotomy, but also feeding gastrostomy. Laryngeal paralysis has occurred in three percent of the living population and eight percent of the deceased. The duration of the tracheotomy has varied from four months to as long as five years in some of our patients before there was sufficient return of function to permit extubation on a permanent basis. The pathology of this problem is not known. There is some relation to the Arnold-Chiari malformation, yet it often seems independent of the degree of hydrocephalus. A few of these patients improve following placement of a shunt, but others, in whom there have been adequately functional shunt systems, nevertheless develop rapid progression of respiratory impairment (Banta et al., 1976). (Suboccipital decompression surgery is being utilized at some centers.)

TREATMENT CRITERIA

Why discuss all of these potential complications or medical problems related to spina bifida? Because it is just such findings that have been utilized by many members of the health professions to present a very negative picture to the young parents and to recommend that the child not be treated, but instead be permitted to die.

There are several large treatment centers across the country, and spina bifida teams are available in each major medical community. Nevertheless, there is a paucity of knowledge presented to the parents at the time of the child's birth. In recent years, a very negative picture has often been painted for the parents. It is important that they receive unbiased information about their child's prognosis and the outcome of the treatment he is receiving, rather than negative input based on obsolete literature and hearsay. It is no wonder that the new parents when first told of this birth defect are overwhelmed with shock, anxiety, and concern about the baby's future. They are torn between wanting to seek the best medical treatment available and conflicting advice by many who tell them that the baby would be better off dead.

Twenty-five years ago, many defective babies were left to die because of a lack of medical techniques for their treatment or because physicians who were not interested in providing such care. This not only applies to spina bifida or hydrocephalus, but to other birth defects as well.

For example, if a child with congenital heart disease also has Down's syndrome, then the advice given the parents might be completely different because of the presence of Down's syndrome and mental retardation sequelae. Many health professionals personalize their own feelings into recommendations to the young parents, so that conflicting advice results. Only in recent years has the patient advocate come forth, and the right of the individual not only to live but to receive optimum treatment has become an important consideration.

In the case of spina bifida, the criteria as to who should live and who should die have come from Great Britain because of the higher incidence of this type of patient in that country. At the advent of socialized medicine in Great Britain in the early 1960s, many reports flooded the literature recommending early treatment with repair of the back defect as soon as possible after birth. Then it was recommended that the children with hydrocephalus be shunted and that the shunts be revised as needed to prevent brain damage due to progressive hydrocephalus or shunt infections, ventriculitis, and/or meningitis. As in any new treatment modality, all types of complications occurred. Many of the children died despite treatment or developed a lifelong disability—a neurological or renal disability being the most devastating.

The burden of caring for this large group of patients upon the finances of the British social structure became evident. This led to an interesting publication by J. Lorber (1971), based upon his study of spina bifida children followed over several years. In his study, he presented prognostic criteria at the initial assessment of the newborn that can be utilized as a basis for selection as to who should be treated and who should be left to die. Lorber's views are illustrated in the following quotation:

> There is no doubt that the future quality of life of many patients with myelomeningocele depends at least partly on the speed, efficiency, and comprehensiveness of treatment from birth onward, and often throughout their lives. Nevertheless, there are large numbers who are so severely handicapped at birth that those who survive are bound to suffer from a combination of major physical defects. In addition, many will be retarded in spite of everything that can be done for them. It is not necessary to enumerate all that this means to the patient, the family, and the community in terms of suffering, deprivation, anxiety, frustration, family stress, and financial cost. The large majority surviving at present have yet to reach the most difficult period of young adult life and the problems of love, marriage, and employment.

It would be of considerable value if one could foretell from simple physical signs present on the first day of life the likely future of the baby if he were untreated, and compare this with his chances if he were given the total care that is known today. Lorber's paper attempted to provide data that may serve as a guide to those called upon to advise and deal with infants born with myelomeningocele. He did comment that it must be remembered that these results relate to older children, whose treatment was not as efficient as would be possible today. Children treated now benefit from the results of several therapeutic trials carried out in earlier years.

Of the parameters examined by Lorber to determine prognostic criteria at initial assessment, four were found to be the most valuable:

1. The degree of paralysis
2. The head circumference
3. The presence of kyphosis
4. Associated gross congenital anomalies or major birth injuries

These criteria were further delineated to select for nontreatment those infants with extensive paralysis at birth, those with a head circumference exceeding the

90th percentile by 2 cm or more, and those born with a gross kyphosis or with major associated congenital defects. In reality, these criteria apply only to a small percentage of children with spina bifida, leaving a vast number in the category of babies who should receive maximum treatment (Lorber, 1971).

Health professionals have lost sight of this, and because of their limited recollection or knowledge of spina bifida, they often advise parents to withhold treatment to almost any child born with a meningomyelocele defect, with or without hydrocephalus or other complications. Often these parents come seeking a second opinion or seeking treatment for a baby two to three months old who did not die, whose head has enlarged considerably since birth, and who now has major complications and deformities as sequelae of failure of early intervention.

If one talks to the physician, one invariably hears that the parents refused treatment. I have never heard a physician say that *he* refused to treat the baby or refused to recommend treatment. There has always been a conflict of reports given by parents and the initial treating physician. Most of the time the picture painted by the initial physician is so bleak—one of mental retardation, severe physical disability, and progressive impairment—that the parents feel that they have the best interest of the child in mind when they go along with such a recommendation. It comes as quite a shock to them later to learn that another treatment course was possible.

Much is belabored about the discussion of the early presentation of the decision to treat or not to treat, because the whole outcome of the psychosocial development of the child and the family can be changed dramatically. A group of professionals met in March, 1980, at Orthopaedic Hospital to discuss the question of whether to treat or not to treat. After a one-day conference of workshops and discussion groups, the overwhelming conclusion was that in the first 24 hours, unless there was some other life-threatening and untreatable condition, the lesion should be surgically closed. This decision was a composite from members of treatment teams throughout Los Angeles County.

Nevertheless, most babies born with spina bifida are not born at the treatment centers, but are usually born in community hospitals and, in one recent case, at a birthing center. They receive varying input of information, depending on the experience of the obstetrician, the consulting pediatrician, or the family practice physician.

The parents, who are already in a stressful situation, should have experienced team members who can knowledgeably present a more positive picture of long-term treatment potential. Ideally, such parents should have access to a multidisciplinary team at a treatment center. When such is the case, the social worker should be involved in the initial discussions with the parents. At our center it is the core team of the pediatrician, the neurosurgeon, and the social worker who usually meet with the parents, either individually or as a group, to thoroughly and carefully explain the disabilities and the proposed treatment plan. Other members of the hospital team may or may not participate in these discussions. During this time, it is helpful if they can be introduced to a spina bifida child and meet with other parents. It is understandable and to be expected that the parents may be in a state of emotional shock. During this time, compounding reality, they are likely to acquire all manner of information, some accurate and some distorted. It is important to answer their questions and to carefully explain the serious ramifications of the birth defect, the systems involved, and the expectations with and without surgery.

Such factors as early repair of the back to prevent meningitis and ventriculitis, early shunting when hydrocephalus becomes evident for prevention of further brain damage, close supervision of the shunt function so that shunt revisions are not delayed to the point of worsening hydrocephalus or shunt complications of infection and ventriculitis—all of these factors can influence the prognosis for the individual child. Later, the early intervention of orthopaedic care; serial casting of club feet; surgical intervention in the case of hip, knee, and foot problems to prevent complicating deformities that may interfere with standing in braces; scoliosis surgery and kyphectomy when indicated; involvement of the occupational and physical therapist to maximize developmental progress; and the progression of standing and ambulation, utilizing braces as needed, will permit the child to attain as normal as possible developmental milestones and will give the parents and the child a sense of normal peer identity.

Early diagnosis of any renal pathology; constant supervision of the GU problems; and prevention of urinary infections, hydronephrosis, and renal insufficiency, which would have a devastating effect on the older child's welfare, are important. All of these factors show the importance of a team approach to the treatment of the handicapped spina bifida child. When all of these services are readily available to facilitate maximum rehabilitation of the child, then the parent can receive positive input and support from such a team and be presented a more hopeful picture of the eventual outcome.

EFFECT ON THE FAMILY

The immediate period following the birth of the child may create many different reactions in family members. One mother, in particular, who had two children with spina bifida, stated that she had been able to respond differently to her children because of the immediate circumstances of their births. Her first child was taken to a nursery immediately following birth, which inhibited maternal-infant bonding. With her subsequent child, they were able to be together for most of the time in the hospital. She said that she has been able to form a closer attachment to the second child because of the manner in which the period following birth was handled. In addition, due to a nine-year time span between the children, she attributed a portion of her positive emotional response to her family's adjustment during that period toward spina bifida.

The initial reactions of medical and other professional staff can either positively or negatively affect parents' subsequent adjustment to the birth defect. One parent reported that she was told not to get attached to her child. During the child's stay at the hospital, the staff would not acknowledge the child's chosen name or use it. The child was later transferred to a facility where the staff presented her with a blunt, yet total, picture of her potential and problems.

The period following birth finds parents asking with disbelief how they may have contributed to the birth defect, as well as denying the possibility of its existence. One father spent most of the time discussing the fact that his wife had an excellent pregnancy, similar to that which produced their earlier, very healthy child. He also emphasized their own medical histories and family backgrounds, in which there was no history of birth defects.

The decision as to whether surgical intervention (closing the sac and shunting if necessary) should be undertaken often needs to be made at a time when the parents are emotionally least able to participate in such a decision. One couple stated that when their child was born, they did not express many opinions or ask many questions because of the feelings of shock they were experiencing at that time. They said later, after taking the child home, that they felt that the physicians interpreted their silence as a desire to let their child die rather than encourage surgical intervention.

Of critical importance to an understanding of parental reaction and to thoughtful and useful intervention is a recognition of the virtually universal grief response that accompanies the diagnosis of the birth of a defective child. This is particularly prominent following the birth of such a child, since the parents mourn the loss of the anticipated, desired, perfect child for whom they had planned. At the same time, they must rapidly adapt to the imperfect and sometimes repulsive child born in its place. Parents experience a major blow to their self-esteem, usually accompanied by guilt. At times they are overwhelmed by the task of withdrawing attachments to the fantasized child, while tending to the ever-present demands of the unwelcome substitute. If they deny their true feelings, they impede the necessary process of grieving and fail to resolve the loss adequately. Mothers are especially at risk, as the infant is generally in their care. Fathers, on the other hand, with their lesser involvement in child care, have less opportunity to become attached to the infant. At the same time, they may feel themselves excluded because of the preoccupation of their wives with the infant.

The necessity and inevitability of expressions of bewilderment, sadness, anger, and disappointment cannot be too strongly emphasized. The parents must allow themselves to experience the range of emotions associated with acute grief in order to proceed with the mourning process. They often need to have the sanction of physicians and other caregivers to permit this to occur. They need recognition of their personal hurt as individuals in their own right, not simply as persons obligated to look after the sick child. A fairly regular observation regarding families of chronically ill children is that of the overwhelmed, overinvolved, resentful mother, and the abdicating father. This distortion of the paternal and marital roles is particularly prone to occur in hereditary disorders, in which resentment about the parent's responsibility for transmission of the disease may poison all but the most solid relationship. Both men and women fear a further reproductive tragedy that may result in a serious disturbance of their sexual relationship, further stressing the marriage. Not uncommonly, marriages fail to survive such strains.

Overprotectiveness is a very common problem with regard to the handicapped child, and this is very evident as the child grows older. A parent often feels guilt at having produced a handicapped child and may overreact by treating the child as younger than its chronological age. Part of this is a normal reaction on the part of parents, since the child with spina bifida often does appear younger because of lack of mobility, incontinence, possible intellectual deficits, and the lack of growth and development of the lower limbs. These factors contribute toward viewing the child with spina bifida as younger than he actually is.

Many problems relating to the care of the child extend beyond the period of infancy. His incontinence necessitates that parents become involved in urinary care, intermittent catheterization, incontinence devices in the young male, and being sure that urinary infections are prevented. Some of these problems, if neglected, can have serious consequences, and for this reason, the parents hesitate to relinquish some of the caretaking to other people or to permit the child to assume self-care responsibilities as he grows older. The lack of sensation in the lower limbs can lead to pressure sores, make the child more prone to burns from hot bathwater or from contact with hot upholstery in car interiors that have been in the sun, and render him vulnerable to other aspects of daily life that would not cause concern in a normal child. Often, the parents' anxieties are related to their child's safety. Caring for a handicapped child often requires more time and effort than caring for other children, and quite often it is much quicker for the parents to do things themselves than to instruct others or delegate the care to the child.

The active treatment period, often during preschool years, produces a number of stresses, as surgery may become more frequent and the child's limitations more obvious, especially with regard to ambulation.

Parents often find it difficult to judge whether it is acceptable or practical to encourage early independence, often because they lack examples of achievement in this area. Also, parents of children with spina bifida maintain protective responses with regard to many life-threatening medical situations, so that it may be difficult to draw an appropriate distinction between reasonable parental responsibility and overprotection.

One parent of a four-year-old expressed concern that she was possibly creating dependency in her child by performing tasks for her rather than letting her achieve the necessary skills on her own. However, she stated that it was often more practical to do things for her child, as it often required less time, which was significant, since coping with a handicapped child presents many time limitations. She also stated that she did not possess the skills she thought necessary in dealing with deficits.

In addition to learning self-help skills, the parents of this child were unclear as to whether she could be expected to have any chores or responsibilities related to family management. The concern was partly due to the fact that she and her husband expected their seven-year-old son to perform certain tasks not required of his sister, and this was creating some hostility in him toward the other family members.

A deliberate policy of involving both parents in responsibility for decisions about the infant from the beginning and of treating them as jointly caring and responsibile enhances their ability to express the many positive aspects of their own feelings for the child. When the parents observe that persons whom they respect express pleasure in the progress the child is making and regard the child not as an object of revulsion but as a child to be enjoyed, they receive renewed strength. Perhaps any faltering in their own self-esteem as parents of a deformed baby is checked when they are treated with respect. Helping the mother secure some form of attendant care or domestic service may be important during the early period in preventing intolerable stress, especially when there are other children, when she is pregnant, or when she is trying to cope with a number of other problems at once. This, too, can help the parents' attitude toward the child and each other.

Children with chronic illnesses and disabilities are at a high risk for developing behavioral and emotional disorders secondary to their chronic condition. A behavioral approach to the treatment of such disorders consists of training the child's parents, teachers, and other careteachers in behavioral management techniques and later in teaching the child self-control skills.

Parents may tend to put less pressure on their children when they are sick or after hospitalization. In such cases the children often regress and insist on more attention. The effects of hospitalization are often a greater source of stress for the parents than for the child, and the reactions of the child depend to a large extent on the hospital setting and the attitude and visiting time given him by the parents. The child with spina bifida may have many hospitalizations for surgical treatment of many of the orthopedic problems related to spina bifida; for treatment of complications such as shunt obstruction, pressure sores, or urinary infections; and for other illnesses that might occur during normal child growth and development. Quite often, repeated operations are done to prevent deformities, and since prevention cannot be seen, the parent and the patient may have a feeling of futility and get discouraged and depressed as a result of repeated hospitalization. With repeated hospitalization, immobilization, and other disease-associated limitations, the individual with spina bifida often finds himself removed from the normal flow of everyday social contact. These episodes, which interrupt interpersonal interactions, may ultimately impede the normal development of assertiveness and social skills, potentially resulting in passivity, mood depression, and a sense of helplessness and hopelessness, leading to even further isolation. This deteriorating interpersonal skills cycle requires vigorous intervention to prevent psychological adjustment difficulties.

Hospitalizations may be numerous for the child with spina bifida; they may be planned or arise due to medical crises. During hospitalization, parents have been observed trying to spend as much time with the child as possible and facing a great deal of anxiety if there are other things to attend to, such as a job or other children who need care. In addition, siblings, especially those who are younger, may experience and express resentment because of the increased time demands required by the child with spina bifida. When siblings are younger, it is often very difficult for them to understand why certain amounts of time are not being spent with them and are being spent with the child who has spina bifida. Because of the presence of the handicapped child, there is often a restriction on family activities. Beyond the day-to-day activities, episodes of illness and treatment can cause further tension and restrict attention for the other child even more. Often these feelings are expressed as jealousy and resentment. Older siblings often react more positively and feel very responsible for and protective toward the younger handicapped child. Both younger and older siblings need information appropriate to their age and explanations of the attention needed for the affected child. Discussion on the part of family and professionals with the siblings needs to be held to deal with the reactions of friends and siblings' unwillingness to have friends over to their house.

From time to time the parents inevitably feel anger because of administrative problems related to their child's handicap, and it is at these times that their patience wears thin. At these times they may appear demanding, aggressive, or ungrateful toward various staff members with whom they come in contact. It is a function of professionals to learn how to accept this, realizing that it is not personal. The venting of hostile feelings is to be encouraged.

PROBLEMS OF THE ADOLESCENT

Development of a sense of identity and achievement of independence are the primary developmental tasks of adolescence (Hayden, Davenport, and Campbell, 1979). Some people think of adolescence as a handicap in itself. Therefore, a handicapped patient going through adolescence has perhaps a double-edged sword, or is in double jeopardy.

Hayden, Davenport, and Campbell (1979) did a study of 49 spina bifida patients between the ages of 10 and 19 years. They concluded that these young people have significant problems, particularly in the area of social function, exhibiting low self-esteem and difficulty with social-sexual adjustment.

It has been noted that adolescents with this physical disability tend to mature earlier physically but later socially and emotionally than their nondisabled peers. In our group of patients at Orthopaedic Hospital, this seemed to be more of a problem in the females than in the males, young girls in the myelodysplasia group showing the greatest emotional disturbance. Older girls expressed more social concerns, particularly isolation and lonliness. Boys had more concern about sexual attitudes and mastery over the environment.

In the study by Hayden, Davenport, and Campbell (1979) it was noted that girls with spina bifida seemed to have had onset of menarche earlier than normal females. By contrast, the males seemed to be behind age-matched controls as a group. Physically, the adolescents and young adults with this defect are smaller than their peers, and many people theorize that this is why some adolescents and young adults give up their braces and remain in a wheelchair. Since their sitting posture is more normal than their standing posture, this choice makes them appear larger than they are.

In an article by Shurtleff et al. (1975) from the University of Washington, the functional status of 98 patients, both adolescents and adults, was reviewed. They, too, found that limited social interaction owing to restricted mobility, embarrassment from bowel or bladder accidents, and realistic concern over sexual adequacy adversely affected psychosocial adjustment, particularly self-esteem. Two-thirds of their patients with normal intellect were functioning as competent adults. However, the remaining one-third were partially or totally dependent upon others for their care.

Self-image is a problem of the adolescent who is undergoing varying developmental changes—some slower than his peers, others at a more precocious rate. Some adolescents normally are concerned if their development is at a slower pace. Others are embarrassed if their development is at a faster pace. Handicapped adolescents have the added impairment of self-image related to physical attributes of spina bifida: primarily paralysis, but also problems related to incontinence, urinary diversion, and the need for incontinence pads or diapers well into a much older age than their peers would expect. They also have a tendency to be more obese than their peers. Some have an enlarged head, as seen in cases of the arrested hydrocephalic or shunted hydrocephalic, and in general may have less desirable physical features overall.

More recent cultural mores have perhaps helped this situation in that adolescents as a group have their unique appearance and dress, so that individuals may have beards or long hair, makeup, or dresses that can conceal some undesirable physical changes. These are all different mechanisms that the adolescent and young adult can use in the present era of social acceptance to camouflage any undesirable appearance. Some of these mechanisms were not socially acceptable in the past. The adolescent should be encouraged to cash in on this trend and develop his own individual characteristics of dress and other means of social expression. Teasing by peers at school is more of a problem for the younger child than for the adolescent. Today it is more of an "in thing" to be different, and the average, normal adolescent is more accepting of the disabled peer.

Exposure may be another problem. The disabled are often grouped in schools limited to the disabled, so that their social contacts are limited. They have much absenteeism from school because of frequent hospitalizations and frequent illnesses, sometimes interfering with their school progress, so that they are often with groups who are younger than they are. This also limits their social exposure and social maturation.

Adolescence can present complex problems in terms of hospitalizations. It is a time when the adolescent may become more fully aware of the nature of spina bifida and its ramifications. The handicap itself may delay the normal stages of adolescence, including aspects of independence, sexual maturity, and vocational plans. In addition, the full impact of his apparent physical differences from other teenagers may reach importance of utmost concern.

Denial of these realities is one way of coping with the differences, and frequent hospitalizations may be the result. Adolescents are often hospitalized with decubiti, which can usually be prevented if one's position is changed frequently. However, if this is not done, the decubiti may necessitate long hospitalizations and, in many cases, surgical intervention. Therefore, when the everyday routine becomes too difficult, a hospitalization may provide a protected atmosphere away from the stresses of life. The hospital may also be one in which other disabled adolescents are present, thereby decreasing the feeling of being different. In addition, a hospital may meet dependency needs. One mother, whose son had been hospitalized frequently, made a request of the hospital staff during a recent admission. She asked that her son not be allowed to return his meals if he was unhappy with a particular one, as he had often done in the past. She felt that this was an inappropriate waste of food and may have been contributing to a desire on his part to be hospitalized.

During several admissions, one teenage lad expressed strong feelings of preferring the hospital to his own home, as he had difficulties interacting with his family, yet he was unable to maintain positive relationships during these admissions with several staff members as well as other adolescents on the same unit.

Social isolation is further fostered by our architectural barriers and transportation problems, which contribute to lack of activities outside the school or the home. The handicapped adolescent has to think twice before he can arrange for a social outing. Both he and his family need encouragement in seeking out-of-home and out-of-school social exposure. Participation in organized events should be encouraged. Wheelchair olympics and other activities are available on an increasing basis. Groups specifically for handicapped teenagers allow them to learn organizational and social skills. The special olympics programs provide an opportunity for competition and success. Previously withdrawn teenagers are now using physical education and after-school time to practice for such events. In the process, they can increase their social contacts and their physical strength and learn that skill comes with practice. Adult role models are important, and contact should be encouraged with successful disabled adults. Sometimes this can be accomplished by employing persons with physical disabilities in the hospital or clinic setting or in the school and by having exposure in the community. Parent and advocacy groups are of particular help in this regard.

In past years, education of the disabled was an isolated experience in special schools and sheltered environments, and only recently has the interest in mainstreaming education emphasized the demand for greater integration with able-bodied peers, encouraging flexibility on the part of schools and educators to enable the disabled pupil to attend regular school. In the past, the special school for the "handicapped" was close to the regular neighborhood school so that the disabled child could participate in some activities or classes part of the day. More recently, the trend has been to encourage complete mainstreaming of the disabled child into the regular school program. This would permit both educational and social adjustments at an earlier age.

In mainstreaming, or placement of the disabled child into what is referred to as the "least restrictive environment," certain effects occur. Positive effects on the disabled child are thought to be improved self image, improved interpersonal skills, increase in likelihood of social acceptance, and the reduction of negative peer and teacher expectations. Possible negative effects on the disabled child would be initial or continuing emotional stress, physical stress, academic difficulty, and social difficulty. When school placement was discussed with disabled adolescents and young adults, they all felt that experience in "handicapped" schools in the earlier years permitted a protected environment and provided important equipment to permit them to develop as many skills as possible. However, as they got older, they felt that a regular school environment was more important and permitted better social contacts and development of social skills. Integration of physically disabled pupils is a complex problem. However, the teenagers with spina bifida when polled, all seemed to be strongly in favor of an educational system that permitted more contact with physically normal peers. Those who had such contacts seemed to have more successful social adjustment skills.

Rebelliousness and argumentativeness are said to be common features of adolescent development. This seems to be less of a problem in disabled patients, as this group of patients has more of a passive personality. They are prone to periods of depression, tendencies to less social activity, feelings of inadequacy, and a propensity to suicidal thoughts. Even though this group of patients cites thoughts of misery and depression and suicidal ideas, very few report any suicide attempts. There is very little in the literature about suicide attempts among this group of patients. Yet, suicide is a serious problem among adolescents in general. Physical limitations and lack of physical access may be factors in the low suicide rate among disabled adolescents.

Adolescents who are still in school express considerable worry about work and opportunities for work as they grow older. Some of these worries may have a foundation in reality, particularly for the more disabled teenagers and for those of below-average intelligence. Access to educational opportunities and work-training opportunities is still sparse. Counseling in this direction is often limited. More opportunities are becoming available for independent living and work training opportunities which are fostered by more successful disabled persons such as organizations for disabled and independent living centers as well as vocational rehabilitation services in the community. Group contact is available for young adults with similar disabilities to share feelings and information about mutual concerns. They are often fearful of seeking advice from parents or health professionals about personal problems and concerns. Rap sessions with peer groups permit interactions that can uniquely support and reinforce the ego of the youthful participant.

DIRECTIONS FOR THE FUTURE

Much has been discussed about advanced medical technology in improving the quality of life and survival for this group of patients. In the past, the focus of medical care has often been on crisis intervention and sustaining life itself. In the future, much of our emphasis can be on improving life.

In May, 1979, Orthopaedic Hospital in Los Angeles began its behavioral medicine intervention for independence program. This is a family-centered bio-psychosocial program designed to maximize individual potential. In this project, behavioral medicine techniques have been utilized by team members who provide a training program for the patients, parents, and family members to help the child attain functional and emotional independence.

Training in behavioral medicine procedures is provided whenever possible to the patient and/or the family in the home setting. The special team has worked with patients and their parents in several specific areas: gait training or walking, weight control, toilet training, and other self-help skills. A group training program for parents helps them to learn behavioral therapy techniques in order to subsequently teach their children self-help skills and manage behavior problems. It is theorized that utilization of these techniques on behalf of the young child will pay off as the child grows older. They will help him cope with growing up and attaining proper social and self-care skills, which are so important in the development of mature, well-adjusted, and independent adults. Some of the future goals for this project include teaching patients greater responsibility for health-related behaviors and discouraging needless dependencies on hospital staff by helping patients reshape their support systems within the family and the community (Manella and Varni, in Press; Killam et al., 1981).

Charlotte Taylor, James W. Varni, and Shelby L. Dietrich (1979) have reported that most chronic disorders and health settings provide a potentially unlimited source for assessment and intervention within the dimensions of behavioral medicine. Performance inventories are used to assess individual self-care levels, enabling the targeting of interventions for specific skill deficits. In addition to such self-care skills as dressing, eating, and grooming, skills are needed in the prevention and treatment of decubiti, urinary tract infections, and obesity (Taylor, Varni, and Dietrich, 1979).

In such areas as decubitus care, urinary tract infections, and exercise programs the interface of the disciplines of nursing and physical therapy with behavioral techniques may result in improved health care services for these potentially serious problems. In addition to teaching such vocationally relevant skills as activities of daily living, bowel and bladder management, hygiene and grooming, and interpersonal relations, the intervention for independence project will apply behavior therapy methods in a training program for adolescents and young adults to facilitate the process of maturation of abilities and interests and to aid in reality testing and shaping of an occupational self-concept. The adolescent and preadolescent years are appropriate times for such intervention. Self-concepts begin to form prior to adolescence, become clearer during adolescence, and are transferred into occupational terms.

The program will provide training in strategies leading to choice of job or field of study and job finding. There are behavioral procedures applicable to job counseling and training programs, that is, self monitoring, screening of alternative choices, behavioral rehearsal, feedback, imitation, and practice in the natural setting. These procedures can be used to teach skills in career decision making and the skills required in job finding (such as job search, interview, organization or resume, etc.). It is then hoped that the adolescents and young adults will increase their independence and participation in the job market (Taylor, Varni, and Dietrich, 1979).

Today there is a far greater sensitivity among the general public to the problems of people with disabilities. It is now accepted that most disabled people must be integrated into the community, and to do this, they must be enabled to achieve the greatest possible degree of independence. Due in part to this growing awareness, the trend has emerged during the past decade to educate children with disabilities in regular schools whenever possible. This educational process is described as "mainstreaming." While many parents welcome the fullest possible educational integration for their children, others feel that their children need the protection of special schooling. Mainstreaming does not signal the end of all special schools, nor should it. There are many severely disabling conditions that preclude a child's being educated satisfactorily in any school that is not geared to meet his speical needs. Yet, study after study has shown that most disabled children who are not mentally impaired do better academically when educated in regular schools than when they are isolated in special schools. Children with certain disabling conditions clearly can adapt more easily to mainstreaming than others. Strong support services are the key to successful mainstreaming. Perhaps the most significant aspect of mainstreaming is the implications it has for a better understanding in the future between the disabled and the able bodied. It has been shown with all minority groups (and the disabled are certainly a minority group) that contact with the community in general during the formative years tends to remove the fear and distrust that lead to later segregation. It seems reasonable to assume that mainstreaming will lead to more open attitudes and more opportunities for the disabled in every aspect of life: jobs, friendships, and every kind of social activity.

REFERENCES

Banta, J.V., Dyck, P., Gilbert, D., Hartleip, D., and Whiteman, S. Review of myelodysplasia. Paper presented at the American Academy of Orthopaedic Surgeons (February, 1976).

Black, P.McL. Selective treatment of infants with myelomeningocele. *Neurosurgery, 5,* 334–338 (1979).

Brocklehurst, G. *Spina Bifida for the Clinician.* J.B. Lippincott, Philadelphia, (1976).

Crandall, B.F. Alpha-fetoprotein: The diagnosis of neural-tube defects. *Pediatric Annals, 10,* 2 (1981).

Hayden, P.W., Davenport, S.L.H., and Campbell, M.D. Adolescents with myelodysplasia: Impact of physical disability on emotional maturation. *Pediatrics, 64,* 53–59 (1979).

Killam, P.E., Apodaca, L., Manella, K.J., and Varni, J.W. *Behavioral Pediatric Weight Rehabilitation in Myelomeningocele: Program Description and Therapeutic Adherence Factors.* Unpublished manuscript, Orthopaedic Hospital, Los Angeles (1981).

Lorber, J. Results of treatment of myelomeningocele: An analysis of 524 unselected cases, with special reference to possible selection for treatment. *Developmental Medicine and Child Neurology, 13,* 279–303 (1971).

Manella, K.J., and Varni, J.W. Behavior therapy in a gait training program for a child with myelomeningocele. *Physical Therapy* (in press).

Patten, B. Embryological stages in the establishing of myeloschisis with spina bifida. *American Journal of Anatomy, 93,* 365 (1953).

Shurtleff, D.B., Hayden, P.W., Chapman, S.H., et al. Myelodysplasia problems of long term survival and social function. *Western Journal of Medicine, 122,* (1975).

Taylor, C., Varni, J.W., and Dietrich, S.L. Behavioral medicine approach to the care of the patient with spina bifida: Intervention for independence. *Spina Bifida Therapy, 2,* 165–194 (1979).

16

The Psychological Effects of Duchenne's Muscular Dystrophy on Children and Their Families

Irene S. Gilgoff

During the course of Duchenne's muscular dystrophy there will inevitably be many inherent stages when the atmosphere seems almost set up for emotional upheaval and family strife. Duchenne's is an ironically tragic disease. At the time in a child's life when he should be gaining in strength and body control, he is losing. At a time when other children are beginning to demand and achieve independence, he, instead, is losing independence. Both the child and parent are painfully aware of the knowledge that he is that way because of something passed on from Mom.

To expect a family and a child to face all this without total dissolution of the family unit or without severe emotional stress seems almost absurd. Yet, amazingly, most families and children do face their life, even with so many cards stacked against them, managing to smile and laugh, managing to cope, If, indeed, there is a question as to the emotional stability of the child with Duchenne's muscular dystrophy and the stability of the family, the more appropriate one might be: How do most of them manage as well as they do?

Duchenne's muscular dystrophy is a sex-linked inherited disease. Genetically, it is believed to have a very high rate of spontaneous mutation, reputedly one of the highest rates of any known disease (Dubowtiz, 1978a). Perhaps some of these spontaneous mutations are actually due to the lack of a truly accurate test for diagnosing the female carrier. Other cases thought to be due to spontaneous mutation might really have had previous family members affected, but misdiagnosed, in the past; for example, a family history of an atypical polio might be obtained on careful questioning. Because of the basic genetic pattern, the child with Duchenne's muscular dystrophy is a boy; the carrier of the trait is his mother.

The boy with Duchenne's muscular dystrophy appears to be a normal child at birth. However, it is known through fetal autopsy studies that the disease process actually begins *in utero* (Mahoney, et al., 1977). The child probably will appear normal until about five years of age. In many families, however, a careful developmental history may reveal that the boy walked late, walked strangely, or

229

perhaps walked on his toes by about three. Indeed, in families with one son with Duchenne's, a second son is often diagnosed clinically by three years of age. By five, the child is usually noted to run slowly. He falls more frequently than his peers. He gets up more slowly. Yet at this age, he continues to try to keep up. It is usually at this time that the boy is first presented to his physician.

Insidiously and relentlessly, the disease continues. The child's weakness originally affects the proximal muscles—those of the hips and shoulders—progressing to a weakness of every muscle in the body. Between 10 and 14 years of age, the boy no longer has the strength to walk and becomes totally dependent on a wheelchair for transportation. In a few more years, the weakness progresses further, to the point where he can no longer brush his own teeth or feed himself. Even control of his head eventually becomes impossible, and his head must be held up by artificial means when he is seated. Families of the older boys frequently report that while their son is riding in a car, his head is uncontrollably jostled around by every turn.

Death, which usually occurs in the boy's late teens or early twenties, is most often caused by pneumonia. The respiratory muscles become too weak to breathe effectively. The abdominal muscles are too weak to produce a functional cough. Death can occasionally be caused by cardiac arrhythmias or by congestive heart failure, since the cardiac muscle is also involved in the general disease process (Perloff et al., 1967; Frankel and Rosser, 1976).

Duchenne's muscular dystrophy is a well-described, fairly uniform disease, with predictable stages of physical degeneration; yet with all that is known about this disease, there remains much that is unknown. What it is that actually causes the muscles to degenerate is unknown (Rowland, 1976; Mokri and Engel, 1975; Cooper, 1977). Also, there is a well-established incidence of intellectual impairment in these same patients (Marsh and Munsat, 1974; Rosman and Kakulas, 1966). Long an area of dispute, it is now believed that this condition is not secondary to the physical disability associated with muscular dystrophy, but instead is another closely linked, genetically determined problem. The mean I.Q. of the patient with Duchenne's muscular dystrophy has been found to be around 85, whereas the mean I.Q. of the normal population is 105 by the Wechsler scale (Dubowitz, 1978b). As mental retardation currently is defined as an I.Q. below 70, it is important to recognize that the majority of these boys, though intellectually impaired, are not by definition mentally retarded. The intelligence curve of boys with Duchenne's muscular dystrophy also follows a bell-shaped curve; however, the peak of the curve is one standard deviation lower than that of the curve of the normal population. It is important to note that, although the muscle weakness is progressive, the mental impairment is not a progressive process.

The purpose of this chapter is to look specifically at how boys and their families deal with the major disabilities associated with Duchenne's muscular dystrophy. Information has been obtained through a search of current literature, which unfortunately is scarce, and also through the personal observations and experiences of several health professionals currently working in this field. In attempting to discuss the psychological effects of so devastating an illness, it must be assumed from the beginning that we are dealing with generalities. Individual patients and families react differently to their situation. Many environmental, social, and economic circumstances will influence their outlook. With this in mind, some general points will be explored.

THE DISEASE FROM THE BOY'S PERSPECTIVE

Ordinarily the child will not look upon himself as ill until parents, friends, and health professionals turn his attention that way. While he is acutely aware that something is wrong, he may not conceive of it as an illness. Probably his first reaction to his problem is one of frustration. Young children so often are judged by adults in terms of their motor achievements. Formal testing such as the Denver Developmental and Gesell tests put heavy emphasis on motor-related activities. When a child first walked is often equated with how bright a child is by parents and professionals alike. In our society the mastering of physical activities is especially emphasized when that child is a boy, a reality that may serve to intensify the boy's feeling of frustration.

The little boy with Duchenne's muscular dystrophy has often been thought of as a normal child until he is five or six years of age. He has competed, with varying degrees of success, as an equal to his peers. With the passage of time, however, his peers gain in strength and coordination. During the same time sequence, he is losing strength; he is more awkward, less coordinated. He cannot win in a foot race. He soon cannot keep up at all. His peers at five and six have mastered a tricycle and are well on their way to conquering the two-wheel bicycle. Most boys with Duchenne's never make that transition. I have only met one boy who was able to accomplish this important milestone. Even with practice, most are unable to succeed. Along with the frustration this produces comes an added sense of failure. Too young to understand why he falls during the race, he is old enough to know that he is not winning.

At this same age, school has just begun. Because of the intellectual impairment seen frequently in this disease, he often finds himself a failure at school also. Again he is unable to keep up; again he is frustrated. On the other hand the boy of high intelligence with Duchenne's muscular dystrophy often will place major emphasis on his intellectual prowess in an attempt to compensate for his failure in physical areas. Even though one might think that this particular child might achieve some form of balance between his successes and his failures, in reality this particular child appears more frustrated by any failures and has greater difficulty in coping.

How the child deals with his unending and deepening frustration is extremely variable. The single most important factor is the atmosphere in his home environment, a rule that seems equally applicable to any child, handicapped or not. The attitude taken toward him by parents, siblings, and friends is the most critical factor in determining the boy's adjustment. The family who accepts their child for what he is, even before the diagnosis is made, takes much of the pressure off the child's shoulders. The family who is equally frustrated by their child's lack of success in the day-to-day competitive world of children adds considerably to the child's frustration.

What happens to the boy emotionally at the time of diagnosis is virtually unknown. Again the family's attitude toward him, and how much they choose to share with him, is critical. The few studies that have been done on boys with Duchenne's tend to agree that the boys who adjust better are those who are dealt with honestly by parents and professionals (Prugh, 1978; Travis, 1976). Answering questions when they are asked and at the child's level of understanding tends to ease many fears. Either refusing to discuss his disease with him or bluntly lecturing on the entire spectrum of his disease before he questions or can understand will cause problems. It is equally illogical to tell a six-year-old boy how many years he may survive as it is to tell him there is nothing wrong. Amid the confusion and the tears of the day of diagnosis, little indeed can be truly hidden.

On a recent morning I had the task of telling a mother of her young son's diagnosis. The mother and I sat alone in a separate room, allowing her time to cry openly before returning to her son's side. After our talk, she wished to be left alone awhile to collect herself before leaving the room. During that time, I took the opportunity to talk to her son in the waiting room, which was crowded with boys in varying stages of weakness and their families. Finding the child, I sat down beside him and briefly explained where his mother was and that she would soon be coming. He was serious, even somber. He did not turn to look at me, only studied in detail the electric wheelchair of an older patient, closely observing as he maneuvered around in front of him. When I asked if he had any questions about his visit to us that day, his only verbal question was, "Who put the (reflector) lights on the back of the wheelchair?" He ventured no other questions.

At best, the day of diagnosis is a confusing time for the child's parents. The boy faces the confusion of his family with equal confusion. He responds to his family's tears with his own concern. Just as the mother feels guilt for what she has "brought upon" her son, so he may feel guilt for the pain he has somehow caused his mother. He may actually feel, too, that his illness is a punishment for any wrong he may conceive of having committed in the past. The only way through this mire of tangled emotions is by a step-by-step building of a road of open communication and trust.

The boy's weakness continues to progress. He returns many times to the clinic to see special physicians, all wanting to help him. The knowledge that he is ill slowly becomes an integral part of him. Some boys have surgery and are placed in braces to aid them in walking. This again draws attention to his disability. Physically and environmentally, his weakness continue to be highlighted, his strengths forgotten. One young boy recently looked down at his withered legs after the removal of his casts following a recent surgery. "I hate this," he said. The nurse close to him stated, "I know it is hard to have casts and surgery." "No, I hate this muscular dystrophy," he replied.

For several more years the boy continues to walk. Eventually, however, his weakness puts him into a wheelchair. He becomes more and more dependent on others for everything, from catering to his physical needs to catering to his emotional needs. As the weakness increases, his social contacts often decrease. Because of problems in lifting him and transporting him, he tends to go to others less and subsequently becomes more dependent on those who continue to come to him. The boy with some intellectual impairment will often be left in a regular school initially, but as his physical handicap increases, he will more commonly be sent to a school for orthopedically handicapped children. This period of transition in his life must be a very difficult one. In general, the boys outwardly assume one of two basic ways of dealing with this stage of their disease: they either become very withdrawn to outsiders or verbally angry.

Bearing in mind that generalizations are dangerous because they can always be proven wrong, the tendency seems to be that boys with higher intelligence show more anger with health professionals as a response to their disease, while boys with learning difficulties become more withdrawn. The boy who at least can continue to compete with his peers intellectually often shows much bitterness that physically he cannot compete and that the physicians who deal with him are unable to change this. He is more resistant to medical suggestions, rejecting braces and wheelchairs until he can no longer fight the inevitable. During clinic visits he is more demanding of his parents, particularly his mother, asking to be repositioned frequently, disputing her decisions or suggestions, constantly correcting her reports of recent respiratory infections or of camp outings. His never ending, underlying question is, "Why me? It's not fair."

The more common reaction to the progression of the disease, however, seems to be withdrawal. Just as physically the child is withdrawn from many outside activities, emotionally he seems to retreat inside himself. The typical patient who comes to clinic rarely speaks. When asked questions, he turns to his parents, usually his mother, to answer for him. If she, in turn, refers the question back to him, he answers shyly and briefly. Some degree of this may be due to the weakness itself and the increasing energy expenditure that it takes to breathe and to talk. Not all of this behavior can be explained this way, though, as other equally involved patients speak up for themselves quite well. Regardless, many boys are quiet with us, withdrawing into withered bodies. Television becomes the major contact the older boy has with forces outside the home environment.

Some families are exceptional. Many mothers tell us that at home the boy continues to be talkative. They have managed to maintain a channel of communication between themselves and the boy, keeping this one external gateway open to him. Even with the increased physical difficulty involved, some families manage to keep the boy participating in family and social outings. With the changing approach toward the handicapped person in society in general, and with today's major thrust toward mainstreaming and continued participation, we may see even greater changes in this in the future. The Muscular Dystrophy Association, with its camp program for children, adolescents, and adults, contributes greatly to this ideal and to the boy's emotional well-being. Most children avidly look forward to these camp experiences and bring home fond camp memories.

In general, the major enduring relationship the boy has is his relationship with his mother. His mother is his protector and usually takes the major responsibility for his physical care. Although it is a relationship frequently charged with guilt, generally it seems to be the most comfortable relationship that he experiences. One recent attempt to evaluate family interactions substantiated this, showing that identifications were strong between the boy and his mother but generally were quite weak between father and son (Siegel and Kornfeld, 1980). This one study showed also that about 25 percent of the boys felt distant from their siblings, perhaps removed from them first by physical barriers, but also by emotional ones.

A close and intricate relationship exists between son and mother. For both participants the relationship is a unique balancing act. Where does protection become overprotection? Where does need become dependency? Each family approaches these problems in a manner distinctly unique. Just as each individual relationship is different from all others, so is each relationship itself changing daily and yearly. Early in the relationship the boy turns to mother for comfort when he falls and injures his knee, but then time passes. Eventually, it is this relationship that the boy comes to count on for fulfillment of almost all of his needs, physical as well as emotional.

The timing of this increased dependency could not be worse. The boy is approaching adolescence when his weakness makes him wheelchair-dependent. Adolescence classically is a time of redefining of parent-child relationships. In the routine scheme of life in our society, adolescence is the time when children begin to break away. The adolescent tries to prove that he is an independent individual with separate likes and dislikes, with separate goals. At the same time, the child's body shows signs of sexual maturity. Often the adolescent becomes painfully modest. He also becomes aware of his sexual desires. Adolescence is, normally, a time of parent-child conflict.

For the boy with Duchenne's muscular dystrophy the conflict is necessarily modified. His desire for independence is overshadowed by his physical dependency. His modesty is confronted with the reality that his mother must bathe him and lift him on and off the toilet. With sexual maturation come new conflicts. Initially, the boy is strong enough to fulfill himself with masturbation. With time, he is too weak even to be able to move his hand close enough to his penis to allow him this release.

The mother-son relationship in the patient with Duchenne's muscular dystrophy is as variable as the mother-son relationship in boys who do not have Duchenne's. At one end of the spectrum is the mother who may conscientiously care for her son's physical needs but is unable to address his emotional pain. At the other end of the spectrum is the mother who is not only aware of her child's physical needs, but is also aware and dealing openly with his emotional needs.

Death is a subject that seems rarely broached. With its glaring inevitability ever present, it still is ignored by many professionals and families alike. Emotionally, how the boy faces this inevitability is virtually unknown. One fact still remains. Each boy's reaction is again individual, varying with family attitudes and religious background, among other things. In general, these young men are well-acquainted with death. In contrast to the relatively sheltered lives of most nonhandicapped children, these boys, by the time they enter their mid-teens, have experienced the loss of classmates and camp friends. Clinic visits can at times reverberate with the talk of another child who has died. Because of this and the association of the hospital visits with past surgeries, return appointments for some boys become a much-feared occurrence. It is not a rare complaint from the family that the boy does not want to come back to the clinic, nor is it a rarity to have the family missing appointments as the boy grows older.

Although dying may not often be an openly discussed issue, it is evident that the boy is well aware of his fate. Our muscle disease clinic follows children with several different diagnoses. Several young men with other medical diagnoses, but with equally withered bodies, have told me of wondering why they had not yet died as they entered their late twenties. Having learned that other young men, with whom they had strongly identified, had died, they had assumed their fate would be the same.

One mother shared with us her son's particular approach to his death. After recuperating from several recent respiratory infections that had come close to taking his life, the boy again became ill. At this point he told his mother that he was tired of fighting and did not want to fight any longer. He said that he was ready to die. The family had previously discussed with him the possibility of tracheostomy and respirator treatment, and the boy had decided against this with the family's support. Although the mother reported that with the end near, it was extremely difficult to honor this agreement, this was done, and the boy did expire shortly thereafter. Retrospectively, the mother was able to discuss this difficult time with the confidence that she and her family were comfortable with their decision. We can only hope that other boys and families are as well-adjusted to this eventuality.

One conclusion that studies have come to is that open communication is essential (Prugh, 1978). All health professionals who deal with patients with fatal diseases such as Duchenne's muscular dystrophy need to be prepared to discuss these issues with the patient and each member of his family whenever this becomes necessary, whenever the question arises. Since the questions are often not asked in a straightforward manner, each member of the health care team must listen carefully to understand what the underlying worry truly is. In discussing issues as sensitive as a patient's own death, one must remember that the greatest tool of any healer is compassion. One must be honest with the patient, yet not deny him hope from wherever the patient finds his hope. Although these discussions may be difficult and timeconsuming, they are of extreme importance, perhaps more important than an injection or a past surgery. The aim of medical treatment of the patient is to prolong life and to make each life as fulfilling and as comfortable as possible. Both at the time of diagnosis and at the point of death, the boy who is most comfortable with his disease is the one who has been allowed to discuss his disease and its many implications when he was ready.

THE DISEASE FROM THE FAMILY'S PERSPECTIVE

Again there is great variability in how parents handle their son's disease. Since this is an inherited disease, many parents have been forewarned of the dangers in childbearing. Some mothers have spent their childhood years caring for their own invalid brothers. The desire to have children, mixed with the fear of completing the hereditary cycle, causes varying degrees of turmoil for each female known to be a carrier of the Duchenne trait. Some women will immediately seek medical intervention and a tubal ligation. Others will mother several children with Duchenne's muscular dystrophy and still continue to have offspring, considering this to be their cross to bear in life, that all this has been predestined for them. Most women caught in this predicament find themselves lost in an area between the two extremes, unhappy with either choice and frustrated with medicine's inability to give precise prenatal information. The state of the medical art at this time is only to inform the mother whether her unborn child is a boy or a girl by a routine amniocentesis. Whether the son is a normal child or an affected one cannot as yet be determined prior to the infant's birth. Thus begins a supercharged game of Russian roulette, and a mother's unborn son's fate hangs in the balance.

The family with no previous history of Duchenne's muscular dystrophy presents a totally different picture. This is a couple anxious to start their family, feeling assured that their sons and daughters will be strong and beautiful. There is no foreboding, no ominous signpost to signal the danger ahead. The delivery of their son is not tinged with fear or guilt; nothing dims the optimism of the child's first breath. The first few years are no different for them than for any other family. (Their child finds success and he experiences failure.) They compare him to the neighbors' and to their friends' children. It is not until the boy is about five years old that they first come to the doctor with their concerns, and then the original complaints are often no more serious than that he is clumsy or awkward. Perhaps the kindergarten teacher sent them because she felt he falls too often. They feel that maybe they are overreacting; after all, he has always been a healthy child. He is hardly ever sick, at least not more than the other children on the block. He even looks strong, his large calf muscles encouraging their fantasy that there really is nothing terribly wrong with their son. They wonder if maybe they are not pushing him hard enough; perhaps he is lazy.

As the process of diagnosis begins, the family's concerns grow. This process will vary somewhat from clinic to clinic. Often the child is referred from the private pediatrician to a more specialized center for the workup. This move alone heightens the parent's anxiety. The family watches as frightened spectators, as the team of specialists examine their son, percussing his reflexes, palpating his swollen muscles, asking them detailed questions about climbing stairs, getting up from the ground, riding bicycles. Blood tests follow; sometimes an electromyogram and even a muscle biopsy are necessary. The shield of denial is weakened as each additional test becomes more complex.

When the family is finally told the diagnosis by the physician, the family again may react in many different ways. Some still are totally surprised. Even the elaborate diagnostic workup has not alarmed them enough to contemplate so devastating a disease. Their son looks too good. For some families the resilient defense mechanism of denial can survive even after lengthy conferencing to explain the child's illness. Several months after an hour's conference explaining the diagnosis to a family, we received a phone call from a therapy center where the boy was being seen. The therapist's request was for a diagnosis, since the family had recently told her that no diagnosis had as yet been made.

Other families, totally unprepared for such unpleasant news, will choose simply not to believe it; often they will consult another physician. It may not matter how much diagnostic proof is made available to the family. For some, even if the diagnosis is heard and expected, the dire prognostications cannot be believed. Often this will begin a never-ending process of shopping from one physician to another, to chiropractors, to naturopaths, or for magical cures with vitamins and health potions.

Anger also is not an unusual response. "Why me? Why us? It's not fair." This anger can be aimed in many different directions. The father can blame the mother. The mother can strike out at her son, her mother, or anyone else available. The family can join together in opposition to the physician. Because of this anger at the diagnosing physician, missed appointments are not uncommon immediately after the diagnosis has been given. The family in a sense is blaming the physician for making the son's illness a reality with his words.

Then there is guilt. This also is a frequent reaction, especially on the part of the mother in blaming herself for her son's predicament. Even without a family history, without any possible way a mother might have known she was a carrier of this genetic trait, some mothers can never forgive themselves. We have had mothers explain to their sons that it is their "bad blood" that is responsible for his problems. Other family members may contribute to the mother's sense of guilt, and not least in this picture is the son himself. Her guilt can be a potent tool he can use against her, if necessary.

Amid all the defense mechanisms is the central emotion—sorrow. From the day of diagnosis the family begins to assess its loss. The parents' dreams and expectations for their son, whether it be college, business partner, doctor, or lawyer, are suddenly destroyed; total reassessment becomes necessary. The father's hopes for a son to play catch with or to cheer on the football field are shattered. The lifelong hopes for social success, marriage, and grandchildren become painful memories. The frightening reality that the parents will outlive their offspring is all that remains.

With all of this, surprisingly, most families survive. Current divorce statistics in families that suffer no major family tragedy are reaching 50 percent and above. To surpass this with a statistically significant percentage would require a very large number of families. In our clinics, families do not surpass the national norm. The family compositions are similar to society in general. Single-parent families, either with mother or father as the remaining parent, are seen. Some families struggle on the verge of divorce, their problems perhaps heightened by the complex special problems they face—and perhaps not. Yet, for each family in trouble there seems to be another one that becomes a more cohesive unit from their shared misfortune. Brief looks at the families of our patients show no shattering statistical difference between them and the average family in our turbulent ever-changing society. We do not seem to be seeing psychopathology in our families. Lifelong patterns of defense mechanisms or individual neuroses present many years before their son's diagnosis remain and may be heightened, perhaps temporarily, but psychosis is very rare. Suicide or alcoholism seems no more prevalent than in society in general, though no detailed studies have been done to fully document this.

In one form or another the family continues forward. Detailed studies of families of children with Duchenne's muscular dystrophy are sadly lacking. The little information that is available does point to a few similarities between families (Siegel and Kornfeld, 1980). As mentioned earlier in this chapter, the central relationship usually is between mother and son. The father more often than not takes on an ancillary role, removed somewhat from his ailing son. Siblings too, are somewhat on the periphery. Part of this shift is due to sheer necessity. The amount of time required to adequately lift, bathe, and care for the growing boy with Duchenne's is prohibitive. Part of the siblings' shift to the periphery of the family, however, is also due to their sense of guilt, fear, and anger. One sister after many years of watching her brother's plight was finally able to profess that she hated to go out to dances because she knew that he could never dance. She felt terrible guilt for her healthy body. The siblings of these patients have much with which to deal. Along with their empathy for their brother is hostility for his position of favoritism with their mother. Mixed with sorrow at his sad fate is anger for his special protected position within the family.

As the boy's weakness grows, the family's defense mechanisms change. Each major change in the boy's ability sends new shock waves through the entire family structure. Diagnosis is followed several years down the line by loss of ambulation. A manual, self-run wheelchair is replaced by an electric one a few years later. Then respiratory failure becomes evident, and the child's imminent death becomes the overwhelming and ever-present issue. The defense mechanism of denial must be discarded. Any defense mechanism that replaces it must be flexible enough to allow the family to meet the increasing physical demands entailed in providing full-time nursing care. The family must work each day for the boy's survival. Inevitably the early years of guilt and sorrow give way to submission, if not acceptance.

New stages in the child's disease process are often faced by the family with a sense of ambivalence. The sorrow of watching the boy sink down irrevocably into a wheelchair is flavored by the relief that they need never again fear his falling uncontrollably to the pavement. The thought of the child's death, too, is tinged with the knowledge that the suffering—the boy's, the family's—will indeed have an ending.

As the boy approaches 20 years of age, his weakness has reached the point of significantly involving the intercostal muscles and the abdominal muscles. The boy's chest expansion is markedly diminished, as is his ability to cough effectively. If surgery has not been done on the back to stabilize it, most boys will also develop a severe scoliosis, compromising even more the already decreased respiratory reserve. Now any respiratory infection can prove fatal.

The choices left to the family at this point are few and universally unsatisfying. The natural course of the disease would be for the boy to become ill with a cold, to progress rapidly to pneumonia, and to die within a few days' time. The family may choose at this time of crisis to care for the boy at home, but more usually will prefer to bring him to the hospital for his care. Just as the years preceding, the last days are relentlessly progressive and agonizing. The boy struggles for breath, and the family watches helplessly. The medical staff too becomes a helpless bystander. Visits may become short and infrequent. The physician too is overwhelmed by the frustration of his inability to change what nature has begun.

Out of these frustrations, alternatives may again be raised. As the patient's lungs begin to fail him, the possibility of using a respirator to assist him is often raised. The decision as to whether to place the boy on a respirator is a multifaceted one. It can only be made with the expectation that he will never be able to breathe again without the use of the machine. The decision, therefore, entails the commitment to a tracheostomy and full-time respirator dependence. The boy's life can indeed be prolonged for many years. There are men currently living on respirators who are now in their middle and late thirties. Yet, medical intervention at the time of the boy's death is just as painfully inadequate as it is in the realm of prenatal diagnosis. The altnerative of lifelong dependence on a respirator cannot offer the family the hope of reversing a degenerative process. It can only offer the possibility of prolonging it. As dismal an alternative as the respirator may seem, when the boy is gasping for air, it also becomes a difficult alternative to ignore. Unfortunately, in the confusion and the desperation of the final days of the boy's life, often these decisions are made with little thought or even with no inclusion of the family and the boy in the decision-making process. Even with years of possessing the knowledge of the inevitability of these final days, the ultimate end often finds everyone totally unprepared.

And what becomes of a family after the boy has died? What irreversible scars have been left on each family member that survives the ravages of this devastating disease? A few families have kept in contact with us even after their son's death. Their mourning process showed no great difference from others who have lost sons or brothers. The boy is grieved for, and fond memories of good times and days of laughter are shared and reshared. The pain too is remembered. Many tears have already been shed and more remain to fall. The son has died, but the grandmother's eyes watch fearfully at each grandson's first steps.

CONCLUSION

Duchenne's muscular dystrophy is a devastating disease. Boys who should grow strong face lives of progressive weakness and early death. Parents who should thrill at their child's growth watch helplessly as their young son dies. Brothers and sisters learn of life's injustices at a very early age. The opportunity for self-pity is obvious; family upheaval is perhaps even to be expected. The experience at our clinic, however, does not confirm these theories. Like families in war zones, life somehow continues and families survive. The health professional working with these boys and their families is privileged each day to be a witness to their unique courage and strength.

A recent study asked several parents of boys with Duchenne's what their greatest problem was in handling their son's disease (Buchanan et al., 1979). Only 25 percent of the families mentioned a physical problem, such as lifting the boy or transporting him. Seventy-five percent of the families felt that some psychological problem was the paramount issue. Families mentioned difficulties in peer relationships, in the boy's isolation and in his lonliness as their major concerns. This study should alert all health professionals to two very important things; one, that as health professionals we should begin to take a closer interest in the emotional status of our patients and their families. For the overall well-being of our patients, this is a major area of concern too long ignored. The second piece of valuable information gained from this study is that our families are way ahead of us in already actively dealing with these issues.

Little still is known about these sensitive areas in our patients' health care; much remains to be learned. Through focusing more attention in this direction and by offering more aid to both the patients and the families more information will become available to us in the future. Yet with all the added knowledge from 100 patients, one thing will remain unchanged: each situation, though linked in a shared tragedy, will forever remain totally unique.

Acknowledgments are made to Carol Alford and Anne S. Gilgoff for their assistance. Special thanks to Dr. Ralph E. Perry.

REFERENCES

Buchanan, D.G., LaBarbera, C.J., Roelofs, R., and Olson, W. Reactions of families to children with Duchenne muscular dystrophy. *General Hospital Psychiatry*, Vol. 1. Elsevier North Holland (1979), p. 3.

Cooper, R.A. Abnormalities of cell-membrane fluidity in the pathogenesis of disease. *New England Journal of Medicine, 297,* No. 7, 371–377 (1977).

Dubowitz, V. *Muscle Disorders in Childhood,* Vol. 16. W.B. Saunders, Philadelphia, (1978a), pp. 32–33.

———. *Muscle Disorders in Childhood,* Vol. 16. W.B. Saunders, Philadelphia (1978b), p. 22.

Frankel, K.A., and Rosser, R.J. The pathology of the heart in progressive muscular dystrophy: Epimyocardial fibrosis. *Human Pathology, 7,* 375–386 (1976).

Mahoney, M.J., Haseltine, F.P., Hobbins, J.C., Banker, B.Q., Caskey, C.T., and Golbus, M.S. Prenatal diagnosis of Duchenne's muscular dystrophy. *New England Journal of Medicine, 297,* 968–973 (1977).

Marsh, G.G., and Munsat, T.L. Evidence for early impairment of verbal intelligence in Duchenne muscular dystrophy. *Archives of Disease in Childhood, 49,* 118–122 (1974).

Mokri, B., and Engel, A.G. Duchenne dystrophy: Electron microscopic findings pointing to a basic or early abnormality in the plasma membrane of the muscle fiber. *Neurology, 25,* 1111–1120 (1975).

Perloff, J.K., Roberts, W.C., DeLeon, A.C., Jr., and O'Doherty, D. The distinctive electrocardiogram of Duchenne's progressive muscular dystrophy. *American Journal of Medicine, 42,* 179–188 (1967).

Prugh, D.G. Why did it happen to us? A psychiatrist explores chronic childhood disability in the family. *The American Families* series. Smith, Kline and French Laboratories, Philadelphia (1978), pp. 1–12.

Rosman, N.P., and Kakulas, B.A. Mental deficiency associated with muscular dystrophy. *Brain, 89,* 769–788.

Rowland, L.P. Pathogenesis of muscular dystrophies. *Archives of Neurology, 33,* 315–321 (1976).

Siegel, I.M., and Kornfeld, M.S. Kinetic family drawing test for evaluating families having children with muscular dystrophy. *Physical Therapy, 60,* 3 (1980).

Travis, G. *Muscular Dystrophy: Duchenne's Form, Chronic Illness in Children, Its Impact on Child and Family.* Stanford University Press, Stanford (1976), pp. 403–431.

17

Psychotherapy for the Physically Disabled Child:
Combining Interpretive/Supportive Therapy
with Behavior Therapy

Claude Amarnick

INTRODUCTION

The therapist's expertise in aiding the physically disabled individual in learning how to cope with his environment cannot be understated. In patients who have suffered a major physical disability, the interplay between physical and emotional states is reflected in the vicissitudes of their rehabilitative course. In about 50 percent of adults with physical disability, emotional and mental factors determine the success or failure of rehabilitation (Rusk, 1977). In children, the figures run approximately 75 percent (Rusk, 1970). It is important to have a knowledge of the patient's earlier life experiences, style, and premorbid personality traits in determining how one can best motivate the patient to cooperate in the rehabilitative program. These developmental factors are of extreme importance because they represent the wide variety of life experiences and situations and the coping mechanisms one utilizes to adapt to his environment. Response to stress during this critical period varies according to what the individual's early experiences have been.

A physically disabled patient, because of the chronic nature of his illness, needs to have psychotherapeutic intervention as soon as possible. A prompt combined treatment approach prevents the development of secondary gain factors, which, if not confronted early enough, would complicate the condition once they have become entrenched.

The therapist must encourage the patient to grieve for the loss of a body part or its function, to go through a process of shock (demonstrated by regression and excessive demandingness, withdrawal and apathy, denial, depression [internal turmoil], anger, and hostile rebellion [external turmoil], and, finally, to reach acceptance through a process of exploring reality and ventilating his apprehensions in an insight-directed psychotherapeutic process. There is a "requirement of mourning" that demands that the patient show proper respect for his loss and for the gravity of his situation. The gradual abatement of mourning occurs following the reconstruction of the body image and self-concept to accommodate changes and the reestablishment of a sense of personal worth (Krusen, Kottke, and Ellwood, 1971).

Depression is always associated with loss and is allied with feelings of grief and mourning. It is not uncommon to personalize the body and feel that it is a cherished possession. Loss of function of a limb or loss of the limb itself is regarded in the same way as the loss of a loved one. The stages of bereavement must be worked out in the same way as one mourns the death of a loved one.

A patient's depression can be treated through ventilation in an interpretive, insight-therapy setting and by use of contingency contract programs, where the patient is able to attain mastery over his environment. The patient should be given significant ways to appropriately negotiate issues over which he can exert control, while the staff sets firm limits in areas that are nonnegotiable. Applying in part the principles of B.F. Skinner, in which an operant (the patient cooperating in physical therapy) is followed by a positive consequence (earning enough tokens or points to have a weekend pass or participate in a special outing), the frequency of positive behavior will increase (Krusen, Kottke, and Ellwood, 1971).

Understanding the psychodynamics and the interrelationship between the adolescent stage of development and body image is of paramount importance. The adolescent struggles for independence and carries his growing body image as a torch and symbol of his quest for autonomy. During adolescence there is a resurgence of psychophysical developmental activity, it is a time when intrapsychic tensions must be reworked and transcended if full adulthood is to be achieved (Blas, 1979). This reactivation of earlier emotional conflicts must be understood in treating the physically disabled adolescent, as well as in understanding the adolescent's intrapsychic struggle with authority figures. Since the body image is integrated with personality organization, such a change threatens the equilibrium of the personality. Physical deformity is usually of great influence in the evaluative self-concept, especially in our culture, which emphasizes physical appearance disproportionately. From Shakespeare's *Richard III* to Pomerance's *The Elephant Man,* literature has constantly reminded us of the importance of body self-concept and how the psyche utilizes this input from the environment.

CASE STUDIES AND ANALYSIS

Case 1

T.L. is a 15-year-old male who had an above-the-knee amputation of his left extremity due to a gunshot wound inflicted upon him by his intoxicated stepfather when T.L. refused to obey his orders. Following the incident, T.L. was taken to the emergency room of a university hospital, underwent emergency surgery, and was placed in the acute care section of the hospital. While there, he received physical therapy for preparation of a progressive ambulation training program. T.L. remained in a state of emotional shock, presenting with a stunned facial expression, a refusal to eat, apathy and withdrawal, and negligible interest or cooperation with the nursing or physical therapy staff. Three weeks postoperatively, T.L. was transferred to the closest long-term pediatric rehabilitation facility, located sixty miles from both the university hospital and from where his parents resided.

Premorbidly, T.L. was described as exhibiting behavior disorders and disciplinary problems at school and at home. Repeatedly, his teachers recommended psychological testing and counseling, but his parents refused, being uncooperative and nonsupportive with the school officials. At home, T.L. often fought and bitterly disagreed with his family members.

The sixty miles from the family home to the rehabilitation facility served as an important physical and emotional distance, removing T.L. from family pressures and allowing him to undergo extensive and intensive psychotherapeutic intervention, along with his ongoing physical and occupational therapies, without the staff fearing parental sabotage. A behavior modification program based on contingency contracts and token economy increments supplemented the interpretive and supportive psychotherapy he received, whereby T.L. learned how to best deal with his greatly altered self-image and restricted independence due to the amputation.

Information obtained during the first few sessions of psychotherapy revealed that in T.L.'s home environment disciplinary measures were based upon the totalitarian beliefs of the stepfather, rather than on a consistent, rational decision-making process where choices and alternatives were available. Repeatedly, his parents had given him negative input regarding his self-worth, causing T.L. to act inappropriately during his lifetime. After obtaining this information, the program instituted at the rehabilitation facility combined behavior therapy techniques with interpretive and supportive therapy. Specifically, the program emphasized allowing T.L. to make choices in structuring the order of activities within his individualized physical and occupational therapy program. The respect and flexibility shown toward him and the impressive gains he subsequently made in therapy greatly added to T.L.'s feelings of self-worth. At all times, however, T.L. understood that important limits were being placed on any inappropriate behaviors he demonstrated and that he was expected to adhere to a consistent therapy regimen. The staff recognized that T.L. was suffering from a major situational depressive disorder, with fluctuating mood swings of withdrawal, apathy, and marked emotional aggressive behavior, and that he was confronting his conflicts of dependence-independence and his regressive processes, associated with mourning the loss of his leg, by ineffectively coping with this object loss. The staff provided support and encouragement within a structured program, thereby demonstrating to him acceptable methods for solving his problems and for giving up his regressive behavioral pattern.

T.L.'s physical rehabilitation program was constructed in conjunction with the recreation therapy department, whereby a token economy system, using a reinforcement contingency contract with timing of reinforcements and privileges, was implemented on a graduated functional basis. When he attended and performed his physical and occupational therapy tasks, T.L. was rewarded by being allowed to attend several recreational activities available in and away from the rehabilitation facility. These activities included movies, visits to nearby shopping malls, concerts, and even being allowed to go to a beach 10 miles from the facility.

From the information obtained from the study of Segraves and Smith (1976), which successfully applied concurrent interpretive-supportive psychotherapy and behavior therapy, it seemed logical to use both techniques in treating T.L. Segraves and Smith's study demonstrated how behavior therapy aided psychotherapy by removing crippling symptoms and giving the patient renewed self-esteem by having him competently manage his daily activities. In the present case, successful behavior therapy elicited changes in T.L.'s attitudes and actions, while interpretive-supportive psychotherapy maintained those changes during his hospitalization and, hopefully, made them long lasting. Segraves and Smith suggest that "psychotherapeutic change in some patients can be accelerated by a two-pronged simultaneous attack on the actual behavior and its internal cognitive mediating events" (Segraves and Smith, 1976, p. 762).

Judd Marmor's (1979) open system of contemporary psychiatric thought helps to substantiate why T.L. made progress. Open-system thinking recognizes that as the patient functions more effectively in a particular area, he gains heightened self-esteem and positive feedback from his environment. Marmor contends that these inner and outward changes modify one's internal psychodynamic system without the necessity of undergoing long-term psychotherapy.

Adolescent developmental issues are closely linked with self-image. An understanding of processes occurring within the adolescent in relation to those images enhances the knowledge of the adolescent's actions. Hauser's (1976) study of adolescent self-images demonstrates how processes such as self-esteem, identifications, projections, delineations, fragmentation, and splitting are relevant to the concept of self-image, since they direct attention to what the individual does to and with self-representations.

Perhaps one of the most important aspects of this comprehensive rehabilitation program was the dramatic qualitative change in which T.L. interacted with his peers. Prior to his disability, he did not possess the required techniques for social interaction and communication on an equal footing with his peers; the use of force was his only form of communication with them. The goal to improve social interaction and develop healthy relationships with his peers was accomplished in the inpatient ward setting by focusing in on the environment and by using group therapy techniques. The ward setting lessened the intensity and strain that one-to-one psychotherapy places on the patient, yet illustrated how he interacted with his peers. The ward setting gave T.L. accessibility to the other patients' intense feelings about their own physical disabilities, thereby lessening his apathy and withdrawal and making him more involved and aware of his feelings toward his amputation. In the ward setting, the use of group therapy and the group format exposed T.L. to peers with spinal cord transections, severe burns and rheumatoid arthritis. During the first few sessions of group therapy, T.L. exhibited apathetic behavior and demonstrated low self-esteem by downgrading his own thoughts and feelings, believing them to be less important than those of the other children in the group.

In the Reckless and Fauntleroy (1972) study on groups, it was concluded that group format increases ego support for those with weak ego and lessens isolation and threat of separation (Reckless and Fauntleroy, 1972). Group format was shown to be an excellent medium to make the patient "affect conscious" by stirring up emotions (Reckless and Fauntleroy, 1972, p. 355). Gradually, the marked apathy and withdrawal seen in T.L.'s early hospitalization shifted to participation and enthusiasm as he learned new ways of coping with life's stresses. As his self-esteem improved, T.L. began to make important contributions to the group and develop better relationships with his peers. He learned new forms of communicating and enjoyed participating in the group's activities within the rehabilitation facility.

Using the data from Abramowitz's (1976) study on the effectiveness of group psychotherapy with children, it was concluded that when group therapy seemed indicated, the feasibility of a behavioral pattern, rather than a psychotherapeutic approach based on psychoanalytic theory, was more effective in decreasing disruptive behavior, increasing social acceptance, and improving self-concept.

T.L.'s unpleasant home environment, with a harsh stepfather exhibiting overt and subtle rejection and a family milieu of disorganization and misunderstanding, necessitated family meetings with the staff and the requirement of family therapy sessions. Unfortunately, T.L.'s stepfather refused to attend these meetings, and only limited success was achieved by involving T.L.'s mother with this program. A complete therapeutic program for T.L. within the rehabilitation facility would have included working through the family's psychodynamics and achieving a more effective communication system within the family.

Upon discharge from the rehabilitative facility, T.L. achieved significant physical and psychological changes in his everyday functioning, adjusting to his amputation and engaging in a normal level of social interaction with his peers. Dispositional planning included T.L.'s returning to his family home and receiving outpatient physical therapy at the university hospital. The mother agreed to have him followed by the outpatient psychiatry department, where his behavior could be monitored and his gains maintained. Although in the past some traditional psychoanalytic theories have characterized adolescence as a period of discontinuity in personality marked by much turmoil and stress, recent studies have not concurred. The more recent studies claim that if an adolescent, such as T.L., demonstrates turbulent and antisocial behavior, then psychological or psychiatric intervention is required. A study by Weiner and Del Gaudio (1976) of adolescent psychopathology points out the changing pattern of psychiatric thought exemplified by Masterson, Offer, and others. This trend of thought states that psychological distress is not a normative feature of adolescent development, that boundary lines between normality and abnormality can be drawn, and that the apparent psychological disturbance in an adolescent progresses into adult disturbances if there is an absence of appropriate intervention (Weiner, and Del Gaudio, 1976).

From the data gathered in this case study, it is clear that the use of various psychotherapeutic modalities is effective, that the modalities complement one another and act synergistically in dealing with the psychological problems related to a patient's physical disability and to his premorbid personality.

Case 2

J.Z. is a 14-year-old male who suffered second- and third-degree burns, sustained over 75 percent of his body, in a garage gasoline and paint fire. He was immediately taken to a burn center of a large community hospital and underwent multiple operations for tangential excision and debridement. During this hospitalization, he presented as a serious behavior problem, being physically and verbally abusive to many of the staff members. His struggle was for control and immediate gratification. Ten weeks after the fire, J.Z. was transferred to a long-term rehabilitation center. A contingency contract was immediately instituted, whereby he was awarded points for attending and making gains in physical and occupational therapy. If the patient accumulated enough points on a weekly basis, he was allowed to go home on Sundays and attend professional sporting events on weekday evenings. Activities attractive to J.Z. were available contingent upon completion of specified units of rehabilitative efforts. Cooperating in physical and occupational therapy was followed by a positive consequence.

The key to J.Z.'s success on the rehabilitation floor was the understanding of the dynamics of a depressed adolescent concerned about body image, manifested by acting-out behavior. The staff was attuned to the extent and type of problems he was confronting and allowed him to ventilate his fears and express his needs for independence. The staff reacted appropriately toward his hostility by using a combination of therapies: interpretive, supportive, and behavior modification. The staff held several meetings to discuss his progress and worked together in a unified, consistent, and rational approach. Many of the programs initiated were concrete enough for him to understand, and he made excellent gains in the range of motion of all extremities, neck and trunk exercises, and in activities of daily living. It was only with the reduction of the grieving process that he began to attach value to the things he could do and experienced reward for the increments in his accomplishments. The key to resolving his grief reaction was arranging events that ensured that he could begin shifting to an achievement-oriented value system for the assimilation of his disability with his future life.

In addition to the staff personnel, two members of the Phoenix Society, a division of the American Burn Victims Foundation, joined in the care of J.Z. The members functioned as role models (both men suffered disfigurement from severe burns during their own adolescence), showing the patient how successful they were at overcoming the disfigurement issue. J.Z. ventilated his feelings of inadequacy with individuals who had dealt with identical issues. The underlying concept of the entire approach toward the patient conveyed that although life was always difficult, it was definitely worth living and should be developed to its maximum potential.

Case 3

F.B. is a 25-year-old male whose T-5 transection of the spinal cord resulted in paraplegia after a motorcycle accident. He was hospitalized in a community hospital following the accident and remained there for four months. Subsequently, he was transferred to a rehabilitation center, where the staff immediately set up a structured rehabilitation program to allay his fears. However, F.B.'s emotional state during the hospitalization was stormy. At first, he refused to attend physical and occupational therapy and presented with an extremely labile mood, switching erratically from a depression about his paraplegia to a state of euphoria in which he believed he would overcome any obstacle and eventually ambulate independently. Upon admission, it was clear that F.B. suffered from an exogenous depression, with use of denial, poor impulse control, and a low frustration tolerance. Clearly, he was in transition in learning to deal with a body that was vastly different from the one before the accident. On further probing, F.B. admitted to anorexia, insomnia, and nausea. These symptoms alternated with episodes of reaction formation, during which the patient claimed that "everything was fine," occasional refusal to attend individual and group psychotherapy sessions, and regressive behavior.

The Grinker and Robbins (1954) concept of field theory points out that conditions that favor regression in the adult will activate infantile responses, with the return of manifestations of a psychological triad of dependency, frustration, and hostility. Understanding the psychodynamics of regression pinpoints the need to supply a patient like F.B. with goals that he can master and help him regain partial control over his life. Replacement of the significant object loss by an adequate sustitute is a necessity; by furnishing him with skills to overcome environmental barriers, the regressive behavior subsided.

Another feature of F.B.'s early hospitalization was his insisting to leave the rehabilitation center, his desire to "want to sleep it off." This is an example, according to Engel, of how people react to a natural disaster, such as an earthquake. In the "shock phase," there is a sense of unreality, which is only gradually replaced by the realization of and a response to what is going on. This behavior is an attempt to insulate and protect against the magnitude of the stress, which is too enormous to handle all at once. Engel found these victims to be stunned, dazed, and apathetic. But when their affects were recognized, they were reported as being associated with fear, abandonment, and utter helplessness (Engel, 1966).

Although F.B.'s denial represented an ego defense against the trauma and a means of maintaining the integrity of the personality, it needed to be surmounted if the rehabilitation program was to be successful. According to Silverman (1968), when affects are sufficiently blocked from emotional expression or from representation in thinking and behavior processes, intense hostile and depressive affect results.

Since there was no immediate or real object toward which his anger could be appropriately directed, F.B. demonstrated his resentment toward his traumatic disability by expressing helpless rage toward the staff through his physical and verbal abuse. According to Engel, helplessness and hopelessness are the affects most expressive of loss of object and damage to the self-image, indicating the greatest degree of disorganization in response to stress and reflecting a giving up. Helplessness tends to develop in the person who is more manifestly dependent on external sources for gratification (Engel, 1966). Understanding the dynamics behind the patient's actions and approaching him with a firm, consistent, and rational manner helps alleviate hostile and regressive behavior. Understanding F.B.'s aggression toward staff members, which primarily served his need for survival and his urgent need to overcome opposition, and how this symbolized his transference responses to hospital personnel proved to be an effective starting point. Gradually, F.B. channeled his energy in more constructive, task-oriented directions within his rehabilitation program. Structure within the rehabilitation program has been found to reduce a patient's tension. A modified contingency contract proved to be effective with F.B. Two- or three-hour day passes outside of the rehabilitation center were used as a positive reinforcement, as was allowing him to participate in wheelchair sporting activities. Whenever F.B. made gains in physical and occupational therapy, he was rewarded with one of these two activities. The regressive behavior gradually diminished, and eventually he discussed the details of the accident with a better sense of reality.

Thus, the psychological management was based upon the premise that the patient's depression could be treated through ventilation in an interpretive-supportive therapy setting and through use of contingency contract programs, through which the patient attained mastery over his environment, which his disability had taken away from him.

REFERENCES

Abramowitz, C. The effectiveness of group psychotherapy with children. *Archives of General Psychiatry, 33,* 320–326 (1976).

Blos, P. *The Adolescent Passage.* International University Press, New York (1979).

Engel, G. *The Psychological Development in Health and Disease.* W.B. Saunders, Philadelphia, (1966), pp. 194 and 208.

Grinker, R., and Robbins, F.P. *Psychosomatic Case Book.* Blakiston, New York (1954), p. 133.

Hauser, S. The content and structure of adolescent self-images. *Archives of General Psychiatry, 33,* 27–32 (1976).

Krusen, F., Kottke, F., and Ellwood, P. *The Handbook of Physical Medicine and Rehabilitation.* W.B. Saunders, Philadelphia (1971), p. 765.

Marmor, J. Short-term dynamic psychotherapy. *American Journal of Psychiatry, 136,* 149–155 (1979).

Reckless, J., and Fauntleroy, A. Groups, spouses and hospitalization as a trial of treatment in psychosomatic illness. *Psychosomatics, 13,* 353–357 (1972).

Rusk, H. *Rehabilitation Medicine.* C.V. Mosby, St. Louis, (1977), p. 270.

Segraves, R., and Smith, R. Concurrent psychotherapy and behavior therapy. *Archives of General Psychiatry, 33,* 756–763 (1976).

Silverman, S. *Psychological Aspects of Physical Symptoms.* Appleton-Century-Crofts, New York (1968), p. 89.

Weiner, I., and Del Gaudio, A. Psychopathology in adolescence. *Archives of General Psychiatry, 33,* 187–193 (1976).

18

A Parent of a Disabled Child Looks at
a Hospital and Its Services

Linda Jefferson

As a health care professional, I had developed a certain view of hospitals and of my colleagues in the helping professions. Hospitals were places where I had earned the right to feel comfortable in the practice of my profession, secure in my skills and the respect of my peers. Becoming the parent of a handicapped child changed this irrevocably, altering my perception of myself, the hospital, and the world in general. Never again would I be the same carefree, self-confident person. It was as if my old self had died and a new self had come into a new world where all the priorities are different.

Most parents of disabled children enter this new world the moment that someone, usually a physician, tells them that their child is not, and probably never will be, normal. For some parents this happens immediately at birth. A problem is present that must be dealt with right away and at a time when parents are least prepared emotionally to be making decisions that will have long-term effects. Often physically and emotionally exhausted from pregnancy, labor, and delivery, they are denied their expected reward—the beautiful perfect child of their fantasies which makes it all worthwhile. Instead, they often must make immediate decisions about serious medical problems and, at the same time, try to love and accept their less than perfect child, while mourning the "death" of their fantasy child. This process of course, is not news to those in the health care professions. It is, however, often news to the parents who do not always understand the dynamics of their emotional turmoil. Without proper professional support and guidance during this process, terrible emotional scarring can occur that can affect for years all members of the family.

For other families, the realization that there is something wrong is a gradual process. Often, doubts and anxieties can gnaw away in silence for a long time as the parents become increasingly aware that things are not going well and become increasingly alienated—from the rest of the family's questions, from inquisitive friends, and frequently from each other—as one or the other or each of them feels that the horrible fear, the secret, is his or her burden alone. Health care providers usually do not confirm these fears until there is a substantial body of evidence. So the parents play a little game, living with their private fears, increasingly isolating themselves to avoid uncomfortable questions or comparisons. Then, when the diagnosis finally comes, initially it comes as a relief. "It" has a name, "it" is something recognized, something that has been dealt with by others.

Much of this initial anxiety can be relieved if the families of high-risk infants are involved in a program of follow-up and screening. While this type of program will not meet all needs, it will do much to dispel the feelings of loneliness and being overwhelmed. If the family has not been involved in such a program before diagnosis, at that time it is essential that a mechanism for continuing emotional support be established. For once the initial relief of having the problem finally identified dissipates, reality hits and the mourning process begins. Unfortunately, health care professionals and health care service institutions tend to deal with the situation with professional objectivity and are not always sensitive to the subjective response of the family. While the parents certainly need to learn to deal with the situation realistically, they do not need, and *do not want,* to be robbed of hope. They must be given reassurance that they are worthwhile, that their child is beautiful and precious and lovable. To deny them this in the name of objective reality is cruel.

In my own experience, I have dealt with both previously outlined situations. My son was born three months prematurely and had many subsequent health problems. I experienced a severe depression concurrent with our fears for his survival. During this time my one hold on hope was my pediatrician, who called me every day and was very patient as I asked him the same questions over and over. When the baby's condition worsened, necessitating transfer to a large university hospital over a hundred miles away, even this link was broken, and I spent many sessions of what seemed like hours on hold, long distance, desperately seeking information about my baby, only to be told finally that, "The doctor is unavailable now and will return your call," which he rarely did. Finally, one day, with no prior preparation, a call came from a secretary informing me that my baby was ready to come home.

At no time during these hospitalizations or his almost immediate subsequent one for pneumonia did I meet or was I contacted by a social worker or anyone else who expressed concern about my adjustment or how I was coping. When, over a year later, a doctor looked at me and said, "Your son has cerebral palsy" the only referral was to an orthopedist for therapy and bracing prescriptions. No mention was made of any support groups or organizations. And when we were enrolled in Crippled Children's Services, an interesting experience that entailed taking in all of our financial records for the previous five years (said my husband, "We haven't even been married for five years"), we acquired a public health nurse, who made two home visits and was able to tell us where we could obtain free immunizations, but little else having to do with the world of the disabled—I mention it almost as a parallel universe that exists side by side with the regular one, but of which so few are made aware.

The disabled have been called "the hidden minority," and unfortunately this tends to be true even among health care specialists, who often have an insular view of their own institutions or specialties. This insularity, which is frequently combined with fragmentation of services, necessitates that the patient and/or family must learn to be aggressive coordinators of their own care, a role for which few are educationally or emotionally prepared. Health care institutions that take a reactive, crisis-solving approach rather than an active preventive approach do a great disservice to both their disabled patients and themselves. Preparing a family of a disabled child to be a well-functioning family unit that remains intact and supportive of each member; that complies with all aspects of care; that raises and educates *all* children to be stable and productive citizens, functioning at the fullest limits of their potential, is a complex and demanding task that begins at the moment of diagnosis and requires the cooperative efforts of all members of the health care team. Immediate and progressive teaching, at an appropriate rate, of all the terminology, procedures, results, and consequences of all aspects of the disability must be done. But there also must be established a resource of sensitive support to whom family members can express their feelings of guilt, anger, fear, hostility, frustration, and resentment.

I, through a television commercial for United Way, learned about the United Cerebral Palsy center with a preschool program and parents' group that provided the support I needed during my son's early years. Later, when Rob attended a school for the orthopedically handicapped, the other parents on the PTA board of directors were my support group. This type of support group can very easily be counterproductive, however, if a negative, rather than positive, dynamic is created. Parents of disabled youngsters, confronted with a barrage of requirements from a seemingly endless stream of professionals, many of whom are perceived either rightly or wrongly as being condescending, demanding, and deliberately understanding, find that a "Them-Us" situation frequently arises. Parents feel increasingly powerless to control their own lives on schedules. Typical reactions for the families are to fight back by rebelling against or questioning even the slightest request, or to get back at the institution by initiating legal action, or to get out by simply withdrawing from service or refusing to comply with the care plan. The desired result is for parents to join the team in planning care and in initiating and implementing positive changes on behalf of their child. Support and cooperation from health care providers can assist parents' groups in assuming a positive and productive direction beneficial to all involved. This, however, requires that those professionals come out from behind the barriers of stereotyped behaviors and attitudes and become personally involved in the world of the disabled. The willingness for health care professionals to become personally involved in organizations dealing with the disabled, to subscribe to publications about, by, and for the disabled, and to give willingly of their influence and organizational skills in support of causes benefitting the disabled can do much to change "Them-Us" to just "Us."

A frequent, unfortunate consequence of having a child with a chronic disability is a continuing subtle erosion of the quality of life of the whole family. Initially, an atmosphere of anxiety and frustration pervades. Frequently there are still major health problems, or the danger of the development of these remains, and in this climate of anxiety even minor illnesses are given major significance. This, coupled with the demands of a highly structured care regimen, can cause a great deal of the family's attention and resources to be focused on the disabled child at the expense of the other members of the family. Brothers and sisters never get music lessons or go to camp. New clothes, trips to the beauty shop, even annual Pap smears are a thing of the past for Mom. Dad's hobby, barbershop haircuts, and so on by the wayside, and if a family vacation can be afforded, often barriers or lack of facilities for the disabled limit choices.

Health care professionals must be aware of a variety of so-called "soft costs" that are a constant drain on finances. Incontinent pads, diapers, extra laundry, stool softeners—most of these are not covered by insurance, nor are they tax deductible. Third party carriers will pay for braces, but not for new shoes to go on the braces, and buying new orthopedic shoes and having them transferred on to the braces can run to three figures in cost—and this must be done every time the child's feet outgrow the shoes. Wearing braces often means wearing special clothes, more expensive "husky" sizes, or expensive special closures or alterations in order to ensure good fit, prevent skin problems, and encourage independence. And forget compact, gas-saving economy cars for families who must have a vehicle large enough to transport a wheelchair. Also, not many families require a baby-sitter for a teenage child, unless that child is disabled. The list of economic drains could go on and on.

More subtle—and even more devastating—are drains on emotion and spirit. Brothers and sisters of disabled children can find themselves being shunted aside, competing unsuccessfully with the demands of the handicapped child at great risk to healthy emotional development. The normal tensions and stresses in a marriage receive added strain from the anxieties and demands of a special child, especially if the partners are in different stages of their "mourning cycle," or if one partner or the other is adamantly resisting progress in their adjustment. Sometimes, unfortunately, families will divide, trying to "place blame" on the other camp and to exonerate their own side from "guilt" for the child's situation.

Emotional crises can arise unexpectedly, triggered by unexpected things—a stranger's offhand remark, a comment about "punishment" or "the will of God" can provoke a sudden irrational emotional response. I remember a beautiful summer day shortly after my son had turned two and I was heavily pregnant with my second child. We had decided to take Robbie to the beach, and he was having a fine time, digging in the sand with his fingers and lying on his back laughing up at the gulls as they swooped overhead. Then, down the beach came a group of children, skipping and giggling and playing among themselves. Robbie's eyes became big and started to shine, and a smile spread across his face, for he was a very happy, loving, social little guy. "Hi there," he called out as they went past. As they skipped right on by he called out, "Hey kids, wait for me!" He began to slowly, painfully, drag himself down the beach on his elbows, trying to catch up. I burst into tears as I envisioned him vainly trying to keep up, always crying out "Wait for me!" as the world passed by.

Of course, at that time I did not realize that by junior-high age he would be independent in self-care and walking around campus with short leg braces and forearm crutches. But that was just one step in the struggle—the day when Rob was age seven and really began to question the "whys" of his condition, his crying and screaming, "I don't want to live this way!"—the day he told me that he always dreamed of himself walking and running. And now the normal self-image crises of adolescence are compounded by the demands and limitations of a physical disability; each crisis brings a setback in the adjustment process. A doctor acquaintance of mine, who himself has a spinal cord injury, confesses that for all his successful practice and professional acclaim, one bowel accident immediately reverts him to a whimpering three-year-old.

How does all this relate to health care professionals, especially those that are institutionally based? I hope that these examples will cause them to evaluate their care plans with a view to possible long-range costs to the family. Be creative in adapting or devising equipment and supplies necessary for care. Cleanable and reusable equipment, rather than expensive hospital-type "throw-aways," can be used. Also, parents should not be so overwhelmed with "things to do" to their child that they never get to relate to him in any way except as a therapist—and sometimes don't relate at all to their other children. The primary responsibility of parents to their children is to parent.

Be aware also of the drains on physical strength and energy of both parent and child that the care of a disabled child can cause. Each voluntary movement by a disabled child requires several times the amount of energy expended by a nondisabled child. Many institutions still contain architectural barriers that limit the mobility and independence of the disabled patient. Bathrooms inaccessible to wheelchairs, inappropriate bathing facilities, and heavy doors are examples of problems that limit self-help and increase frustration. Also, be aware that most activities involving disabled children are *slow*. When a disabled child has a doctor's appointment, Mom doesn't just grab her purse and yell, "OK, jump in the car and let's go!" Loading and unloading child, wheelchair, and crutches; braces on and braces off—all these things take time. Health care professionals must understand this and allow each child enough time to do as much for himself as he can, while still being supportive in those areas where he has not developed skill. This requires taking a detailed history from both parent and child in order to learn what skills the child has and to plan for teaching in areas of need.

Well-established continence programs can go by the wayside during a hospitalization. This is usually upsetting to the child and increases his emotional stress, especially if care personnel are not helpful and supportive. While a hospitalization can give an opportunity to review and assess the family situation and the disabled child's ongoing care plan, it is usually best not to add to the child's insecurity by making extensive changes during his hospital stay, unless there is a situation that is threatening to the child's health and well-being. Any care plan developed must be based on the family's situation, lifestyle, and needs, and not on the artificial environment of the hospital. A care plan suitable in a controlled, structured setting may not be possible in the child's home, and if the care can not be fitted into the family's life, there probably will not be compliance with the plan.

The milieu into which an ill child is placed has a great effect on the course of his condition. This is especially true of a disabled child, whose limitations of movement and, often, of communication make him especially vulnerable and, thus, extremely anxious and fearful. A calm, accepting, low-key approach is even more essential than usual, and especially so if spasticity is present. Attempts to rush or sudden or loud voices will increase spasticity, in itself painful even when no surgery is involved. Special assistive devices, soft-touch call lights or bells, communication boards or aids—all will increase the child's feeling of security and his sense of well-being, increasing his emotional as well as physical comfort. The adjustment process to a physical disability is a long-term one with relapses or regressions. When a disabled child faces a health or emotional crisis, he regresses —and so do his parents. Each time my son has surgery, the cold, hard lump in my throat is as large as it was the first time. Do not assume that because a family "has been through this many times" it will be easier for them. This is not true!

Earlier I mentioned the "mourning process" that begins for parents at the moment of realization that their child is disabled. This process involves the whole family, eventually including the child himself as he becomes aware of his disability. In spite of the adjustment process, there still is a constant emotional overlay—some call it a "chronic sorrow"—that pervades a family with a special child. Thus, no matter what the disability, each of these families shares this common bond.

I have continually referred to the "adjustment process" or "adjustment," though the last stage of the "mourning process" is supposedly "acceptance." I do not have acceptance and I never will. Acceptance, from "to accept," means "to take what is offered willingly." While I love my son deeply and am very proud of him, I will never stop sorrowing that he is not tall and straight and strong like his brother, and every parent of every disabled child I know readily acknowledges that he would give up anything—even his life—if his child could be "normal."

Is this unhealthy? I don't think so. To me accepting means sitting down and willingly taking what life throws at you. Adjustment means making the best of your situation, but always fighting to improve it. (As you may have guessed, my most common "regression" on the "ladder" is anger!)

What do I want for my son? I want what other parents want for their children—a normal life. What do I want for my son? I want it all!

INDEX

Abuse, sexual. *See* Sexual abuse
Academic testing, 97
Achievement tests, 97
Alpha-fetoprotein, 210
Amniocentesis, 175, 210
Anencephaly, 209
Antianxiety agents, 16
Antidepressants, 13-14
Antimanic drugs, 15-16
Antipsychotic drugs, 14-15
Apnea, infant, 75
Approach behavior, 31
Aqueduct stenosis, 211
Arnold-Chiari malformation, 211
Arthur Adaptation, 65
Asphyxia, neonatal, 75
Attachment, 24, 46
  approach behavior with, 30-31
  at birth, 46
  of infant to mother, 30-36
  signalling behavior with, 30-33
Attachment behavior, 31
Attention deficit disorder
  with hyperactivity
    antidepressants for, 13
    antipsychotics for, 15
    stimulants for, 11-12
    symptoms of, 12
  without hyperactivity, 12
  residual state, 12

Bayley Scales of Infant Development, 63-64
Behavior rating scales, 7, 96
Behavior therapy for disabled child, 243-251
  case studies and analysis, 244-251
Bender Visual Motor Gestalt Test, 98
Birth, 45
  alternate room for, 47-48, 52-53
    nursing considerations in, 55-57
  education on process of, 47

[Birth]
  history of child's, for school records, 95
  at home, 48-50
  at hospital, 46-47, 51
Bonding
  maternal, to infant, 23-30
  paternal, to infant, 41-42
Breast-feeding, 45-46
  of cleft palate infant, 205
Cancer, 189-196
  diagnosis of, 190
  dying from, 194
  emotional impact of, 189-196
  initial treatment of, 191-192
  prediagnosis of, 189
  relapse of, 193
  remission of, 192-193
  surviving, 195
Caretaking behavior, 31
Cattell Infant Intelligence Scale, 64
Caudocranial dysostosis, 212
Cerebral palsy, 70
  from hydrocephalus, 76
  from neonatal asphyxia, 75
Child abuse. *See* Sexual abuse
Cleft lip
  feeding difficulties with, 205
  hereditary implications of, 204
  multidisciplinary approach to, 201
  surgery for, 206
  treatment of, 203
Cleft palate
  clinic procedure for treatment of, 205
  coordinator in team care approach to, 201, 202
  evaluation of, 202, 204-205
  feeding difficulties with, 205
  hereditary implications of, 204
  psychological considerations with, 201-207

[Cleft palate]
psychosocial treatment of, 203
specialists involved in treatment of, 201
with spinal defects, 212
surgical, dental, and speech treatment of, 203
Clinical child psychologist, 85, 86
Cognitive skills, 89
assessment of, 97–99
Conduct disorders, 12
antidepressants for, 13
Congenital amputation, 183–184
Congenital anomalies, 179–181
Conners Teaching Questionnaire, 96
Craniofacial anomaly clinics, 182
Cystic fibrosis, 176

Denver Developmental Screening Test, 64
Depression, 1, 244
antidepressants for, 13, 14
Developmental disorders, 12
antidepressants for, 13
antipsychotics for, 15
Developmental Test of Visual-Motor Integration, 99
Devereux Elementary School Behavior Rating Scale, 96
Diagnostic and Statistical Manual, 3, 6
Down's syndrome, 213
Draw A Person Test, 100
Duchenne's muscular dystrophy, 229
in adolescence, 234
child development with, 231–234
clinical course of, 229–230
dying from, 235
genetics of, 229
mental retardation with, 230
mother-son relationship in, 235
withdrawal with progression of, 233–234
Dyslexia, 96

Education, 89–90
of child with spinal defects, 223, 225–226
classes, 92
learning disability and, 96
new directions in, 93
special, for exceptional students, 92

Education for All Handicapped Children Act, 93
Educational therapist, 105
Emotionally disturbed children, 105
classroom behavior of, 106, 111
hospitalization of, 105, 107–108
schooling with, 108–112
peer group relations of, 106–107
pleasure principle of, 106
psychoeducational programs for, 105–112
residential treatment centers for, 105
Enuresis, 13

Facial palsy, 212
Family
of disabled child, 253–259
involvement of, in psychotropic drug usage, 8
involvement of, at time of delivery, 53–54
perspectives of, on Duchenne's muscular dystrophy, 236–240
Father
bonding of infant to, 41–42
in child rearing, 42–44
of child with genetic disorder, 184
interaction of, with child, 41–44
treatment of, for sexual abuse, 155

Genetic disorders, 173
child and adolescent development with, 177
chronic illness from, 176–178
congenital anomalies with, 179–181
crisis intervention for, 185–186
despair from, 177
fear and anxiety over, 174
hemoglobin in, 174
hemophilia, 197
hospitalization for, 176, 177
metabolic diseases, 174
phenylketonuria, 178
psychological effects of
on child, 176–181
on parent, 181–186
reproductive attitudes with, 174–175
Gesell Scales of Infant Development, 64

Hearing, 94
  loss of, 95
Hematologic illnesses, 189-196
  diagnosis of, 190
  dying from, 194-195
  emotional impact of, 189-196
  initial treatment of, 191-192
  prediagnosis of, 189
  relapse of, 193
  remission of, 192-193
  surviving from, 195
Hemophilia, 197
  adolescence with, 198-199
  child development with, 198
  diagnosis of, 197
  psychosocial aspects of, 197-199
Hospital services for disabled child,
    253-259
Hospitalization
  of emotionally disturbed children,
    105, 107-108
  for genetic disorder treatment, 176,
    177
  for sexual abuse, 167-172
  for spina bifida, 220, 222
House-Tree-Person Test, 100
Hydrocephalus, 76
  with neural tube defects, 211
  surgical shunting with, 212, 213
Hyperactivity
  antidepressants for, 13
  antipsychotics for, 15
  with attention deficit disorder, 12
  signs suggestive of, 70
  stimulants for, 11-12
  symptoms of, 12
Hyperkinetic reaction of childhood,
    12

Illinois Test of Psycholinguistic
    Abilities, 99
Incest, 119
  endogamous, 120
Incest carrier syndrome, 117
Individual Educational Plan for handi-
    capped, 93, 100
  parental disagreement on, 101
Infant
  attachment of, to mother, 23, 30-
    36
  high-risk, 61-77

[Infant]
  [high-risk]
    clinical uses of evaluation of,
      67-68
    delayed development of, 69-71
    examiner in evaluation of, 62-63
    handicaps occurring to, 75-77
    instruments in evaluation of,
      63-65
    interfacing evaluation of, with
      institutional protocol, 74
    providing feedback to parents on,
      68-69, 71-74
    purpose of evaluation of, 61
    teaching child development, 68
    testing of, considerations in, 65-67
    time for evaluation of, 62
  maternal bonding to, 23-30
  paternal bonding to, 41-42
  premature, 71
  very small, 75-77
Intelligence tests, 98
Intercourse, incestuous, 119
Interview, diagnostic, 6

Laboratory studies, 7
Language, 96
  tests on, 98-99
Language disorders, 70
Laryngeal paralysis, 212
Learning disabilities, 93-102
  assessment of, 94-100
    academic testing, 97
    behavioral ratings and observa-
      tions, 96
    cognitive, 97
    developmental and educational
      history, 95-96
    perceptual testing, 98-99
    physical, 94-95
    social-emotional, 99-100
    specialty testing, 98-99
    speech and language, 98-99
  definition of, 93-94
  educational determination with, 101
  Individual Educational Plan, 100-
    101
  psychological issues of, 101-102
Leiter International Performance Scale,
    65
Lithium, 15, 16

Mainstreaming, 223, 225–226
Mania, 14
McCarthy Scales of Children's
        Abilities, 64
Meningocele, 209–210
Meningomyelocele, 210
    in adolescent development, 220–224
    family affected by child with, 216–
        220
    future of, 224–226
    genetics and incidence of, 210–211
    mental capacity with, 211–212
    psychological considerations of,
        209–226
    treatment criteria for, 213–216
Mental retardation, 15, 76
    with Duchenne's muscular dys-
        trophy, 230
    with spina bifida, 211–212
Merrill-Palmer Scale of Mental
        Abilities, 64
Methylphenidate, 10
Minimal brain dysfunction, 12
Mother
    attachment of infant to, 23, 30–36
    bonding of, to infant, 23–30
    of child with Duchenne's muscular
        dystrophy, 235
    of disabled child, 183
    of spina bifida child, 216
Mother-child interaction, 23–37
Muscular dystrophy, 176
    Duchenne's. See Duchenne's mus-
        cular dystrophy

Neonatal nurseries, 55, 57–59
Neural tube defects
    alpha-fetoprotein levels with, 210
    hydrocephalus with, 211
    incidence of, 210
    orthopedic deformities with, 211
    paralysis with, 210–211
Neurological exam, 94
Night terrors, 16
Nurse, 62
Nurse practitioner, 62
Nursing considerations in delivery of
        infant
    in alternate birth room, 56–57
    in neonatal nursery, 57–59
    with rooming-in of mother, 59–60

Oedipus complex, 136
Oncology illnesses, 189–196
    diagnosis of, 190
    dying from, 194–195
    emotional impact of, 189–196
    initial treatment of, 191–192
    prediagnosis of, 189
    relapse of, 193
    remission of, 192–193
    surviving, 195
Parents. See also Mother; Father
    of child with chronic illness, 177
    of child with cleft palate, 203–204
    of disabled child, 182, 183, 253–259
    of high-risk infant, providing feed-
        back to
        assessment of readiness, 72
        assessment of readiness for
            referral, 72–74
        type of information, 72
    of mentally retarded child, 181, 184
    of phenylketonuria child, 178
    of spina bifida child, 216–220
Parents United, Inc., 155
Peabody Individual Achievement Test,
        97
Peabody Picture Vocabulary Test, 99
Pediatric psychologist, 79–87
Pedophilia, 120
Perceptual testing, 98
Phenothiazines, 10
Phenylketonuria, 178
Physical examination
    for diagnosis of disorders, 6
    for diagnosis of learning disabilities,
        94–95
    of sexually abused child, 169
Psychoeducation, 94
    for emotionally disturbed children,
        105–112
Psychologist
    in assessment of high-risk infant, 62
    clinical child, 85, 86
    as consultant, 83–86
    in HMOs, 84
    pediatric, 79–87
    in pediatrician's office, 80
    in providing feedback to parents, 69
    psychodiagnoses by, 80
    in psychosomatic illness assessment,
        81

Psychopharmacologic agents, 11–16
  antianxiety, 16
  antidepressants, 13–14
  antimanic, 15–16
  antipsychotics, 14–15
  stimulants, 11–13
Psychotherapy for disabled child, 243–251
  in adolescence, 246
  case studies, 244–251
Psychotropic medication, 1–17
  antianxiety drugs, 16
  antidepressants, 13–14
  antimanic drugs, 15–16
  antipsychotics, 14–15
  historical perspectives, 1–5
  major tranquilizers, 14–15
  minor tranquilizers, 16
  principles in use of, 5–11
    baseline assessments, 7–8
    comprehensive evaluation of child, 5–7
    drug selection, 9–10
    drug-free trial and reevaluation, 10–11
    family involvement, 8
    school involvement, 8–9
    titration and monitoring, 10
  stimulants, 11–13
Pupil Rating Scale: Screening for Learning Disabilities, 96

Reading, 90–92
Respiratory distress syndrome, 75

Schizophrenia, 14
School, 8, 9, 89
  academic testing in, 97
  child development in, 89–90
  for emotionally disturbed children, 106
  involvement of, in psychotropic drug usage, 8–9
  psychoeducational programs in, 105
  teaching of reading in, 90–92
Secretary-Boss Test, 100
Separation anxiety, 13
Sexual abuse, 115–172
  behavioral associations with, 144
  definition of, 119–120
  deviant behavior in, 143

[Sexual abuse]
  diagnosis of, 171
  emergency room procedure for, 167–172
  hysteria from, 134
  indicators of, 144
  legal tests in evaluation of, 170
  long-term effects of, 116
  medical history with exam for, 169
  medical tests with exam for, 170
  motivation behind, 120
  neurosis in, 135
  Oedipus complex and, 136–139
  offender in
    assessment of, 124
    fixated, 120–122
    regressed, 122–125
    rehabilitation of, 125
    patterns of, 120–125
  physical exam for evaluation of, 169
  physical trauma from, 145
  projective testing of, 139
  protocols for evaluation of, 145–146
  recognition of, 116, 133
    clinical, 143–146
    psychodynamic deterrents to, 133–143
  role of child in, 125–133
    disclosure, 129–132
    entrapment and accommodation, 127–129
    helplessness, 126–127
    retraction of complaint, 132–133
    secrecy, 126
  scope of, 117–119
  statistics on, 117–118
  treatment of, 146–148, 167–172
  treatment programs
    for anxiety and sleep disturbances, 171
    for injuries, 170
    for pregnance prophylaxis, 171
    for venereal disease prophylaxis, 171
  victimization process in, 118
Sexual assault center, 167–172
  emergency room protocol, 167–172
  personnel, 167
  physician in, 169–171
  social worker in, 168
Sickle cell anemia, 177

Signalling behavior, 31
Social worker, 168
Spina bifida, 209
  in adolescent development, 221
  cause of, 210
  education of child with, 223
  genetics of, 210
  hospitalization for, 220, 222
  hydrocephalus with, 211
  incidence of, 210
  mental retardation with, 211–212
  orthopedic deformities with, 211
  paralysis with, 210–211
  psychosocial adjustment to, 221
  social isolation with, 222
Spinal defects, 209
  anomalies with, 212–213
  in adolescent development, 220–224
  effect of, on family, 216–220
  future of, 224–226
  incidence and genetics of, 210–211
  mental capacity with, 211–212
  treatment criteria for, 213–216

Stanford-Binet Intelligence Scale, 64
Stimulants, 11–13

Teacher
  of emotionally disturbed children,
    108–112
  involvement of, in psychotropic drug
    usage, 8–9
Tourette's syndrome, 14, 15
Tranquilizers
  major, 14–15
  minor, 16

Uzgiris and Hunt Ordinal Scales of
  Psychological Development, 64

Valium, 16
Vanguard Child Sexual Abuse Treat-
  ment Project, 155
Vision, 94

Weschler tests, 65, 98
Wide Range Achievement Tests, 97